Advance Praise

"Our feet are the foundation for the entire body and Dr. Tumen does a brilliant job at helping us put our best foot forward. *Ask The Foot Doctor* offers clear and simple advice that can help kids; athletes to senior citizens understand and overcome an array of foot issues. If you're looking for answers, this book is definitely a step in the right direction."

–Dr. David Friedman
TV & Radio Health Expert
and #1 best-selling author of *Food Sanity*

"Dr. Tumen 's book *Ask the Foot Doctor* should be mandatory reading for anyone wishing to gain knowledge of the beauty and wonder of the foot and ankle. It is full of useful information for any nurse, parent, coach, athlete, diabetic, and anyone wishing to stay or become more active.

This book will save people from the many sources of misinformation about the foot and ankle currently given in social media. It's not only a great reference, but it's an entertaining read as well."

–John F. Grady, DPM
Director, Foot and Ankle Institute of Illinois.
Scientific Chairman, Midwest Podiatry Conference

"*Ask the Foot Doctor* is a great new book for the general public. Dr. Tumen outlines the most common foot problems so that everyone can understand. It'll be a valuable resource for those looking for quick and practical answers."

–Amol Saxena, DPM
Past-President American Academy of Podiatric Sports Medicine

T0163824

Ask the Foot Doctor

ASK THE FOOT DOCTOR

Real-Life Answers to Enjoy Happy, Healthy, Pain-Free Feet

Dr. DOUG TUMEN

NEW YORK

LONDON • NASHVILLE • MELBOURNE • VANCOUVER

Ask the Foot Doctor

Real-Life Answers to Enjoy Happy, Healthy, Pain-Free Feet

Published in New York, New York, by Morgan James Publishing. Morgan James is a trademark of Morgan James, LLC. www.MorganJamesPublishing.com

ISBN 9781642791983 paperback
ISBN 9781642791990 eBook
Library of Congress Control Number: 2018908355

Cover Design by:
Christopher Kirk
www.GFSstudio.com

Interior Design by:
Chris Treccani
www.3dogcreative.net

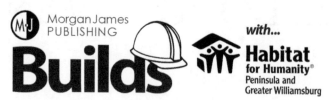

Morgan James is a proud partner of Habitat for Humanity Peninsula and Greater Williamsburg. Partners in building since 2006.

Get involved today! Visit
MorganJamesPublishing.com/giving-back

To Jack and Liza—
the loves of my life.
To Jenna—
For your unending love, support and inspiration.

Table of Contents

Preface   "So, Doc, What about That Book?"   ix

About Hudson Valley Foot Associates—HVFA   xi

Introduction   xiii

Part 1   **Foot Fundamentals: Everyday Care and Prevention**   **1**

Chapter 1   Your Fantastic Foot   3

Chapter 2   "One Shoe Can Change Your Life"—Cinderella   7

Chapter 3   Babies, Toddlers, and Kids: So Grows the Tree   13

Chapter 4   The Fashionable Foot   19

Chapter 5   Fun and Games: Prevent, Prepare, and Play Like a Pro   25

Chapter 6   Seniors: Feet Don't Fail Me Now   31

Part 2   **Your Foot and Ankle: Conditions, Causes, and Cures**   **39**

     "Can I Ask You a Question?" A Guide to Part 2   41

Chapter 7   Fungus Nails: There's No Fun in Fungus   45

Chapter 8   The Ingrown Nail: Cutting Corners   55

Chapter 9   Plantar Warts: Gone Viral?   63

Chapter 10   Bunions: Beyond the Bump   71

Chapter 11   Hammer Toes: Bent out of Shape   81

Chapter 12   Morton's Neuroma: You've Got Nerve   95

Chapter 13   Plantar Fasciitis: The Real Deal about Painful Heels   105

Chapter 14   The Achilles: A Hero of a Tendon   119

Chapter 15   Ankles: The Twists and Turns   129
Chapter 16   Broken Toes: Let's Set Them Straight   143
Chapter 17   Arthritis: A Joint Effort   149
Chapter 18   Diabetes and Your Feet: Time to Team Up   159
Chapter 19   Gout:A Royal Pain   171
Chapter 20   Surgery: What You Need to Know   181
Conclusion   How to Become a VP—Virtual Patient   187

Fun Foot Facts   191
Acknowledgments   193
About the Author   197
Shoes That Fit   199

Preface
"So, Doc, What about That Book?"

When Barbara Neuman first came to the office twenty years ago with a foot problem, she told me she liked my "Foot Facts." These were brief articles about common foot issues that I wrote for the local paper. They ran in a column and consisted of a picture and a blurb about a particular foot topic.

I was pleased that Barbara had read the foot facts and that they had led her to seek treatment at our office, but she told me they could be more. She thought the foot facts could be a book—that I should write a book about foot problems because I had a knack for explaining. She said she should know because she was a technical writer for IBM. I was flattered—what author wouldn't be?—and I tucked the idea away. Years passed, and whenever Barbara came in to have her feet treated, she wouldn't leave the office without asking, "Have you started writing that book yet?"

Then one day, Barbara showed up for her appointment with a file. It was full of all the newspaper articles I had written. She said I had better get going on the book because people were waiting for all the helpful information I had to share. That got to me—the idea of being able to touch more lives and benefit more people. So I took the file and I went home and I began.

Barbara continued to nurture the book and together with her siblings, Dave Neuman and Cyndy Patrick (both editors), gave me expert feedback and kept me motivated as I wrote the first draft. I thank them all for our fun and productive Monday meetings and for being so generous with their time, professional skills, and talents.

What you now have in your hands is my labor of love: the answers to the questions my patients ask most often, the explanations they have found most helpful, and the advice and tips that have encouraged them to improve, not just their foot health, but in many cases, their overall health and well-being. I have witnessed patients change their entire lifestyle to a healthier one. Just the other day, my patient Louise came in for an appointment because she had developed a painful bunion and wanted to have it fixed. She hadn't been in for two years and was so excited. She had lost 75 pounds since I had last seen her. She said it was my consistent urging and belief in her ability to change that made her commit to losing the weight. What a privilege to be a part of her transformation!

I am fortunate and grateful to love what I do. My patients continue to inspire me every day, and I have included many of their stories in the book. Some patients, like Louise, even graciously allowed me to use their real names. They were eager to share their experiences with you. So here it is from all of us to all of you, three decades of foot doctoring condensed into one book for you and your feet. And your feet sure deserve the attention. By the time you are fifty, your feet will have carried you the equivalent of twice around the world. Now, that's a foot fact!

About Hudson Valley Foot Associates—HVFA

G rateful and lucky. These are the words I feel when I talk about Hudson Valley Foot Associates, the place I have called home for over thirty years. I am grateful for so many things about HVFA, but especially for my amazing partners. Our philosophy has always been to do whatever it takes to make our patients happy and pain-free, and to improve their quality of life. I am also lucky because my partners are among my closest friends. To be able to go to work and enjoy what you do with the people you work with is truly a gift. So, for that, I am most thankful.

None of this would be possible without wonderful patients who have put their trust in us and continue to refer their friends and families to HVFA. I remember when I first decided to move to Kingston, New York, in 1986. I grew up in a busy neighborhood on the south shore of Long Island. When my mother first came to visit, I could see the worried look on her face. She asked, "Are you sure you want to practice here—where are the people?" It made me chuckle, but she was concerned about how could I possibly be successful in such a small community.

Mom, the patients came, and thankfully they haven't stopped coming. We at HVFA are so fortunate to be able to serve our patients and our communities. HVFA has now grown to nine offices in seven counties all around the beautiful Hudson Valley. Many of our patients and their families have been coming to us for thirty years now, and we continue to welcome new patients to our practice on a daily basis. It is a bustling and happy place indeed.

Let me introduce you to my partners in podiatry here. Meet Dr. Michael Keller, Dr. Danny Longo, and Dr. Cliff Toback. Three amazing people and amongst the finest podiatrists and foot surgeons anywhere. Dr. Keller is the brilliant surgeon, best I have ever seen. There is nothing he can't fix. He has dedicated his career to academics and teaching. He has served as Residency Director for over fifteen years, training the next generation of podiatrists to be skilled surgeons. Dr. Longo is the doc who does it all. Surgery, wound care, fractures, you name it. He sees more patients than anyone could ever imagine, and gives each one special care and attention. In addition to the practice, he has dedicated himself to the young kids in our community and coaches and leads teams in soccer, lacrosse, and flag football. Dr. Cliff possesses thirty years of experience and is an accomplished do-it-all foot doctor, from surgery to senior care and everything in between. He is beloved by his patients and is blessed with gift of instantly putting a smile on anyone's face. Dr. Cliff spends his weekends either on the lake or the ski slopes. All the docs have fantastic families, great kids, and active lifestyles. We also take pride in our outstanding associate doctors, Dr. David Kim, Dr. Andrew Hune, and Dr. Amanda Maloney. All talented and exceptional doctors.

I often boast about our incredible staff. At HVFA, you will always see cheerful faces. From our exceptional nurses to our administrative staff, the billing department, and our front office team, they are all warm, friendly, and dedicated to making HVFA a great place to be.

A special thank you goes out to Bud Walker, our practice administrator. Bud has allowed all of the docs at HVFA to focus on one thing and one thing only, quality patient care. Bud and his amazing team handle all the daily challenges of a medical practice, so we get to do only what we love to do; take care of our patients. Thank you, Bud, we are grateful for you.

Should you ever visit us, you will be warmly welcomed into our HVFA family. Please call anytime or visit us online at *HVFA.com.*

Introduction

B ecoming a foot doctor may seem like an odd career choice to a lot of you, but it was a natural one for me. My parents gave me two options from the time I was a child: "You can be a lawyer or a doctor." My older brother, Michael, became a podiatrist and loved it. He was always my role model and mentor, so when it came time for me to choose, I followed in his footsteps and chose podiatry.

What I noticed whenever I visited Michael's office was that his patients were thrilled to see him and they left the office joyful, almost walking on air. They loved that the doctor was helping them get past their challenges and back on their feet. I saw that podiatrists have a lot of one-on-one interaction with their patients. That appealed to me. Foot doctors are in hospitals some of the time performing surgery, but mostly they are in their offices seeing patients. That doesn't get boring or routine because podiatric patients present great variety and challenge. Within a day, a podiatrist sees many different problems: a patient hobbled by heel pain, a diabetic with a foot ulcer, a runner who wants to train for a marathon, a senior who just can't walk or care for his or her feet. It seemed like a good life and a great profession, helping people. As a podiatrist, my brother became part of the fabric of his patients' lives. They knew they could count on him to help relieve any foot issue they may have. Everyone in the office was happy, the staff, the patients, and my brother.

There was another strong influence on my career decision. I was and am a runner. It is a passion of mine. I remember the amazing feeling the first time I ran in Central Park alongside hundreds of other runners on their daily run. I was hooked. My passion eventually took me to the starting line of nine marathons including the New York City Marathon, which I completed seven times. There is no more electric feeling than running through the five boroughs of New York, passing about a million cheering fans, and experiencing the thrill of a lifetime as you cross the finish line, completely exhausted, with tears of joy and elation.

The rise of podiatry in the 1970s actually coincided with the boom in running and growing popularity of road races and marathons. As more and more people became runners, there were more foot injuries and more people in need of professional treatment. I realized that helping fellow runners and other athletes with sports injuries would be an extension of my practice, and a "running podiatrist" would be welcomed by the running community.

So I became a foot doctor. And discovered the real deal about feet. People don't think their feet rate. Compared to the big issues that require a doctor's care like hypertension and cancer and cardiac disease, foot problems seem so small. Most people just don't feel their big toe hurting warrants a visit to the doctor. But they're wrong.

Your feet matter! Whatever your age, your occupation, your gender, your feet need attention. They are how you get around and they deserve respect— your respect and your doctor's. Your challenges should be heard and addressed, whether you have aching feet, painful heels, injured ankles, bunions, or hammer toes. Every issue should be given time and consideration.

That's what our practice at Hudson Valley Foot Associates offers our patients. Attentive listening, clear and full explanations, a complete list of options, and a plan for moving forward. We want patients to leave our office with all their questions answered, knowing that together we are going to get them over their difficulty and back on their feet. At our offices, we want happy patients because they feel well cared for, educated, and relieved about any issue they may have. We want them to leave feeling "up."

The response has been tremendously gratifying. I started with a solo practice in Kingston, New York, in 1986 and now, over thirty years later, Hudson Valley Foot Associates serves seven counties in the Hudson River Valley with nine offices and eight doctors. I am also a regular guest on a call-in radio program, Northeast NPR's Medical Monday. I suspect the host Alan Chartock initially invited me because he had a foot problem, not necessarily because he thought podiatry was a hot topic.

The first time I was on the show, I remember sitting in the "on air" room praying the phones would ring and worrying that no one would call in. I even had friends on the ready to call in if necessary. To everyone's surprise in the radio studio, the phones began ringing off the hook for the foot doctor. My podiatry hour continues to be the most popular of the medical specialties. That's because people are eager for a chance to ask all those foot questions they've been putting aside or thought were too trivial to go see a foot doctor about. Everyone has a foot problem of some sort they want to learn about or get rid of.

I want you to have that chance too. To ask the foot doctor any questions you have and get clear and complete answers. That's what this book is for. I want parents to have answers about their kids' feet, teachers and nurses and waiters to get answers about their painful feet, and everyone to know the dos and don'ts of pedicures and nail polish. I want to answer your questions about warts, bunions, heel pain, toenails, tendonitis, ankle sprains, arthritis, and gout. And I want to answer your fears about caring for the diabetic foot. From babies to seniors, from blisters to ulcers, from heel to toe, I want you to ask questions and get answers!

I also want to encourage you to take care of your feet. Good habits can be tough to start. Most of us don't pay much attention to what we should be doing until we're in a bind. But I want to give you the opportunity to be different. To take your feet into your own hands—what a picture!—and start caring for and respecting them before problems develop. So the first part of this book is dedicated to answering basic care and prevention questions: How does my foot work? How do I tell if a shoe is right for me? When should I take my kid to the podiatrist? What are the best nail care practices? How can I avoid sports or weekend warrior injuries? What do I need to know about caring for senior feet?

The second part of *Ask the Foot Doctor* is devoted to exploring common problems. Some of these conditions you may have due to no fault of your own. You can thank your mom and dad for a lot of your foot issues. And circumstance for some. How did you know there was a wart virus lurking in that shower? And you can thank time for others. Everything changes with time, including feet. So if you currently have a foot issue, don't spend time kicking yourself. Skim the table of contents for the chapter on your condition and get answers to these questions: Why do I have this condition? Are there any home remedies I could try? What options will a podiatrist offer? Do I need to have surgery? What are my risks?

Have an issue or a question not covered in the book? Please pursue it! Visit *askthefootdoctor.com* for more details on conditions and treatments. If you are in the Hudson Valley, make an appointment at one of our office locations (at *HVFA. com* you will find our office contact information and more about our practice). Or if you're not in New York, see the Conclusion of this book for a special invitation to become a VP—virtual patient through the magic of telemedicine!

Part 1

Foot Fundamentals:
Everyday Care and Prevention

Chapter 1
Your Fantastic Foot

Did you know that every single day, you are being supported and propelled by "a masterpiece of engineering and a work of art"? That's how Leonardo da Vinci described the foot. Da Vinci produced the first anatomical drawings of feet, and his studies of the mechanics of the mighty foot made him the "pioneer of podiatry." His artist's eye and inventor's mind marveled at both the foot's function and beauty.

Sooner or later, many of my patients end up admiring their feet too. Patients are fascinated when I show them an x-ray of their foot for the first time. "Is that *my* foot?" they ask, utterly amazed by the glimpse of its inner workings. The detailed architecture of the foot is truly an extraordinary sight to see!

The foot is elegant but also highly complex, even when compared to other parts of our body. The thigh has only one bone, the femur. The lower leg has two bones. But the foot has 26 bones.

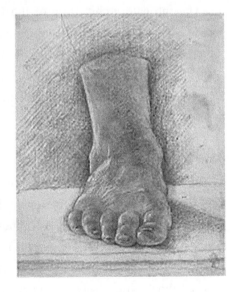

Together, your two feet comprise 25 percent of all the bones in your body. And everywhere there is a bone, there is a joint, 33 in each foot to be exact. Throw in 19 muscles and 109 ligaments, and you realize your foot is truly the work of art honored by da Vinci.

The foot's extremely detailed structure is why podiatry has its own medical colleges and course of study. These provide the time and focus necessary for students to truly understand the foot's design. In most medical programs, students start learning about the body at the top (the head) and work their way down. Often the course time runs out as instruction reaches the feet, so many medical students receive only the most cursory introduction to them.

My most vivid memory from medical school is entering the lab for the first time with my classmates. That day was the beginning of a yearlong exploration of the foot's anatomy. All 160 of us were nervous but soon forgot our anxiety as we became fascinated by the foot's marvelous intricacies. We studied with amazement each delicate nerve coursing through the foot, the hard-working tendons that extend from muscles and attach to the bones to provide mobility, and the tight ligaments that hold each bone together for support.

Why do feet have such a complex design?

The intricate architecture of the foot is required for our feet to do their job. We are descendants of hunters and gatherers. Humans are not stationary structures on stationary foundations. We don't have wings. We have feet. We walk and we run. Our feet must provide shock absorption, stability, and leverage as they guide us over all kinds of terrain. Each and every part of the foot plays an important role.

Your Shock Absorbers

Most of us walk with a heel-to-toe gait. This means when we take a step, the heel is the first part of the foot to hit the ground. It takes the full impact of each step, which is up to one and a half times a person's weight. So if you weigh 100 pounds, your heel may experience 150 pounds of impact with every step. You can figure out what that means when carrying those extra pounds. The arch also absorbs shock with its elastic and supportive abilities. Some arch structures do this more efficiently than others, but we'll talk more about that later in Chapter

2 when we discuss shoes. And, of course, the balls of your feet must provide stability and shock absorption as you propel forward to take the next step.

Your All-Terrain Vehicles

Muscles, tendons, ligaments, and bones stabilize the foot and keep it moving forward and in the right direction. Many tendons extend from the leg directly into the foot, and many more start in the foot and pass through the arch. All work in unison as parts of an intricate system. They function in sync much like an orchestra playing beautiful music. Toe muscles support and balance us as we roll forward onto the balls of our feet. Remember we aren't always walking on an ideal surface. Our foot muscles must adapt to stabilize us over all kinds of terrains: hills, bumps, holes, rocks, ice, and twisting trails.

Your Lift

The foot essentially functions as a lever. The toes are the lever's fulcrum, lifting our body weight to the next step. We move from heel to toe—starting with shock absorption and mobile adapting to the final action, which is called toeing off. All toes play a role, but the big toe is the leader, the star. It does the heaviest work as our foot finishes its liftoff and propels our entire body forward.

How many reps?

Now let's consider how often your feet take you through this heel-to-toe action. Devices that count steps are popular today, so you may even know how many steps you are taking daily. An active person may take as many as twenty thousand steps a day. Even someone minimally active may take between three and four thousand steps between getting up in the morning and going to bed at night. Impressed? And how often do your feet get a day off? So you take thousands of steps, maybe even tens of thousands, seven days a week, fifty-two weeks a year. That's a lot of work. Let's just say your feet deserve much more attention and respect for the hundreds of thousands of successful takeoffs and landings.

Maintenance for my feet—really?

The foot may be an engineering wonder, but no part of the body is designed to last forever. The goal is to have strong functioning feet for as long as we possibly can. Achieving this goal takes attention and care, a lifetime of it. Would you drive a car on worn-out tires or never balance the wheels? We take care of our cars because it's pay now or pay more later if we don't provide the necessary maintenance.

Too many people pay a price for ignoring their feet. Here's the thing: you don't have to. That masterpiece of engineering is your foot! Every day you can make a choice to either abuse or take care of your feet. I hope this book helps add life to your feet, and your feet help you enjoy and discover the beauty of our world. You are the proud owners of two miracle machines and amazing works of art. Your feet are your foundation. It's time to take a stand for them!

Chapter 2

"One Shoe Can Change Your Life"— Cinderella

---

n 1991, a couple of hikers in the Italian Alps found the body of a man frozen in the ice. They thought he was an unfortunate hiker who had met with a fatal accident a year or two before. Well, they were wrong. The man they found was a hunter who had died from an arrow wound some 5,200 years before. Scientists named the man Ötzi, removed him from the ice, and began to study him. Because Ötzi had been frozen, his body was well preserved and so were the clothes he was wearing and . . . his shoes.

Ötzi's shoes were made of animal hide and had a surprisingly sophisticated two-part design, an inner part and an outer. The inner part was a grass net filled with hay, which served as insulation or cushioning or both. A prehistoric insole! The outer structure had a thick sole with extra strips of hide attached to the bottom. Yes, treads! These helped the shoe to grip slippery terrain. The outer shoe had a shank that covered the ankle and a string that tied around it for stability. Ötzi was a hunter surviving in a rugged, harsh terrain, and he wore

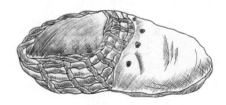

shoes designed to protect his feet and enhance their function. Ancient wisdom from this five-thousand-year-old man.

Exploring Our New Concrete Jungle

Although you may not hike the Alps on a regular basis, the terrain you traverse every day is just as demanding and threatening to your feet, maybe more so. Sidewalks, malls, big box stores, schools, office buildings, factories, they all offer your foot an unyielding, unforgiving, and often painfully hard surface—concrete.

In the scheme of civilization, concrete is relatively modern. Cement was first invented in 1824, and the first concrete street was built in Ohio in 1891. Our ancestors mostly lived on soil and the earth's more accommodating surfaces. We have transitioned over the millennia from hunter-gatherers to the agricultural revolution, and we are now smack dab in the middle of the industrial revolution. We are among the first generations living in this hard, unforgiving concrete world. And we are not doing so well. The evidence of wear and tear is all around us with people undergoing joint replacements to their hips and knees at record rates. And our feet are not happy about it either!

The shoes we choose are all that comes between us and our concrete world. Do you or anyone you know work forty or more hours weekly on your feet—in retail, manufacturing, hairstyling, nursing, or any other profession that requires standing? Do you do this work week after week, month after month and year after year? We may not have a choice about the floor surfaces where we are employed, but we do have a choice about what we put on our feet. And what we wear on our feet may even accelerate pain and the aging process. Unfortunately, all too often we may make poor choices at young ages when we cannot imagine long-term consequences.

Jason is a patient of mine. He manages a retail store, typically standing on his feet for sixty hours a week. His shoes were the classic men's dress shoes with thin soles and a pointy, narrow toe box. His chief complaint was "really painful feet." Although he was only twenty-seven, his feet and body were feeling the effects of standing long hours on concrete, and his joints were aging rapidly, far ahead of schedule. He had arthritis in his knees, painful feet, and a slipped disc. Of course, as a manager he wanted to dress the part. However, every body is different, and Jason's is not designed for our concrete world. Presently, he is wearing better shoes with custom orthotic inserts to diminish his pain. He is also keeping an eye out for a position with a different job description, one that is easier on his body. He understands now that if he keeps doing what he is doing, his later years are going to be saddled with pain and difficult to enjoy.

Your feet are your foundation. Your entire structure depends on them. If the foundation of a building is unsound, you may not want to live in it. It's the same with your feet. If your feet aren't functioning properly, then everything above is going to be affected, from your ankles to your knees, your hips, your back, even your neck. It's miserable to have your feet hurt and have to stand on tired aching feet all day that also make the rest of you ache too. You can help your feet and improve your foundation. Invest in "good" shoes.

How do I Choose Good Shoes?

Somewhere along the line, the shoe lost its most important purpose, to protect and support our feet. Shoes became objects of fashion, designed to be stylish and attractive. Unfortunately, the shift from function to fashion wreaked havoc on our feet. The convergence of concrete and fashion, as we saw in Jason's case, often leads to prematurely painful feet and even permanent damage.

We are often obligated to wear certain styles of shoes. Employment and fashion are not going away anytime soon. So do your best to make good choices and show your feet some love by giving them a comfortable, cozy place to live. Here are four tests and a couple fit tips to make sure you get the best shoes for you.

The Pinch Test

Place a finger on each side of the heel of the shoe. Pinch the sides of the heel together. A good shoe usually has a supportive heel counter. If the heel can be squeezed together and your fingers touch, the heel counter is too soft. Firm is best for support.

The Accordion Test

Hold the shoe between your hands from heel to toe. Try to fold the shoe in half. If it folds in half easily, it does not offer good support. A firm shoe or one with a little bend is best. Think firm, avoid flimsy.

The Sponge Test

Hold the shoe between your hands from heel to toe. Twist it from side to side. If it twists easily, it may make your feet shout.

The Wiggle Test

Your toes should have some room to "move about the cabin." Too tight, not right. Your shoes should fit comfortably upon purchase. And please realize breaking them in is not going to make them feel better. Usually if they are not comfortable in the store, they only get worse when you bring them home. As much as you may want to emulate Carrie Bradshaw, if you find a sale on Christian Louboutin's, best not to squeeze your size 8s into size 7s even it is the most beautiful shoe you have ever seen.

For the best fit, shop for shoes later in the day. Feet may swell from carrying us through the day's activities, and even slight swelling can make a difference in fit. Also note that our feet do change sizes over our lifetimes. Have your feet measured at the shoe store to see if it may be time to move up to a larger size. Comfy feet are happy feet.

What if I can't give up fashionable shoes entirely?

I know those good-for-you shoes won't always win the day against fashion, so here are some tips to reduce the stress on your feet:

1. *Have at least three choices of comfortable shoes in your closet: a good pair of walking or running shoes, one go-to dress pair that is übercomfortable, and a pair of supportive sandals for summer. (Flip-flops and thin-soled sandals may be pretty, but they are hard on the feet.)*
2. *Replace shoes frequently. Many people wear their shoes way too long because they are comfortable (like an old couch) and we fall in love with*

our favorites. When you wear your shoes too long, the shock-absorbing materials wear out. Don't wait until you can play peekaboo with your shoe before you get a new pair.

3. *Give yourself a fashion shoe schedule and stick to it. Wear comfortable shoes to work three days a week and stylish shoes two days. You'll feel the difference.*

4. *Wear supportive shoes when you are going to be on your feet for a long time. Going to Disneyland? Wear good sneakers. Walking a mile on sidewalks to your office every day? Pack your dress shoes and put them on when you get there. Going shopping? Leave the dress shoes home.*

I'm wearing good shoes, so why do my feet still hurt when I'm on them all day?

As we've seen with Jason, some occupations take their toll. Nursing, teaching, retail, and many other professions require standing on your feet for long hours daily. Even with good shoes, people suffer with foot pain. If your feet hurt after a day at work, orthotics may be a solution; they are for many people. Orthotics are customized inserts worn inside your shoes to help eliminate foot pain. I wear mine every day, run in them, and prescribe them frequently to help my patients reduce or eliminate their foot pain.

Why do orthotics work?

Although the foot is a marvelous machine, it comes with imperfections. One example is a flat foot. These feet are often too flexible and tend to roll in, which leads to fatigue or pain. Feet with high arches tend to be rigid, poor shock absorbers, and also frequently painful. Custom orthotics are designed to modify abnormal foot function and eliminate pain. Podiatrists are experts in understanding the inner workings of the foot. We design custom orthotics to change how the muscles, tendons, and bones carry out their repetitive tasks. Subtle changes from abnormal to more normal function can relieve pain, and protect feet from excessive wear and tear.

To fit you for custom orthotics, a podiatrist takes cast models of your feet and works with a professional laboratory to design the prescription appliances specifically for you. This is similar to how an eye doctor prescribes glasses that correct imperfections in your vision. Robert, my patient who is a US Mail carrier, relies on his orthotics to keep his feet free of heel pain. He says just one day without his miracle orthotics and he has terrible heel pain, is hobbling, and unable to deliver the mail on his daily nine-mile route. Whether you are a runner, postal worker, corrections officer, mechanic, or child with tired feet, good shoes and custom orthotics can keep you on the move through rain,

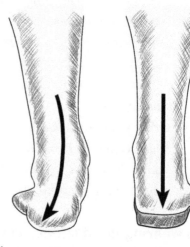

snow, and mostly over miles of concrete. Ötzi would approve! Or as Cinderella would say—if the shoe fits, you'll live happily ever after.

If you are curious about orthotics or would like more shoe recommendations, visit our website at *askthefootdoctor.com.*

Chapter 3

Babies, Toddlers, and Kids: So Grows the Tree

L ittle feet. Remember when your first child was born? What an amazing joy, exhilarating experience, and a once in a lifetime feeling! Did you rush to count the ten little fingers and toes, making sure they were all there? Do you still have their first footprint from the hospital? How small and cute those feet were. Isn't it hard to imagine those now size 10s were ever so tiny?

I remember when Jack, my first child was born. It took me only seconds to inspect his feet, count his toes, and wiggle them around. Was I an overbearing podiatrist already? One of the first things doctors look at is your baby's feet. Are they normal? Is there a clubfoot? Even a baby's first stick and poke for a blood-screening test comes from the heel. Ouch! Welcome to the world of painful feet.

It wasn't long after birth that Jack's feet were "turning in," a condition called *metatarsus adductus*. Even before walking, his tiny feet and legs ended up having weekly serial castings to straighten his feet. He went on to walking straight and became a star on his high school track team, and now his big feet wander the country looking for great photographs. Of course, he wears good shoes and orthotics, and his feet are now eerily similar to mine.

Liza, my second, unfortunately went through a similar process for her feet. She still in-toes just a bit, but her feet are much better than if they had not been treated as an infant. She also excelled in sports but lost her senior high track season to foot surgery after the hurdles got the best of her foot.

We as parents want every part of our child to be perfect, and it can be quite scary to not know if your baby's foot is normal or not. From the time our children are babies until they are young adults, they will present us with foot issues that inspire lots of questions. Below we will tackle some of the most common.

So when do I worry? Will they outgrow this or that as the pediatrician reassures me, or should I get a second opinion?

Babies at birth are screened, and if there is a concern, your pediatrician requests a consultation with a specialist. Thankfully, the most serious foot conditions are quite rare. A clubfoot, for example, is a severe deformity that requires early intervention and usually surgical correction. Incidence is about one in a thousand and is easy to recognize. It will not be missed.

Things get trickier when you get home and have plenty of time to study and inspect every part of your baby's body. Are the legs too bowed? Are the feet turning in? These are questions to bring to your pediatrician, and if there is any concern, the smart thing to do is to get your baby looked at by a specialist.

There are too many adults walking around with foot issues that could have been mitigated with early treatment. That's why Jack and Liza both had treatment even before they were walking. They had correctable issues, and because the bones and soft tissues were amenable to castings, they were dealt with early. It is always sad for me to tell the first-time mom who is attempting to be a great parent by bringing her three-year-old in with a foot problem that she's missed the window for early intervention. Once children are walking, some issues are much harder to correct.

So when in doubt, get a second opinion. All pediatricians want the best for your kids. However, their most common answer to questions about feet is, "Your child will probably outgrow this in a few years." And for many conditions that is correct. But for others, it isn't. A quick opinion from a specialist can confirm that your concern is "no big deal" or identify a challenge that requires early treatment to ensure the long-term health of your child's feet.

When should a baby begin to walk?

Most babies begin walking somewhere between nine and twelve months. A delay is not a concern unless your child gets to about eighteen months and is not walking. Any concerns over motor skills or delays in development should be noticed by your pediatrician and referred to a pediatric neurologist.

Is it normal for a baby not to have an arch?

As your baby begins to walk, not having an arch is not a problem. It is quite common for the feet to look "fat and flat." Arches develop usually by age three and sometimes a bit later. If by age five you can't see an arch, a specialist consultation is probably a good idea.

What about "toeing in"?

This issue is a little tricky because there are a variety of possible causes. Toeing in, or what is commonly referred to as "pigeon-toed," is not uncommon for a child up to about eighteen months or so. If however, toeing in causes tripping over the feet, the child should be evaluated. If a child by age three or four is still toeing in excessively, best to have a specialist consultation.

My child walks on her tiptoes—is this okay?

Lots of kids walk on their toes. It is not unusual as long as they can also walk on their heels. Most who walk on their toes do so out of habit and will correct themselves over time and with a little encouragement. On occasion the Achilles tendon or the calf muscles are so tight that the heel cannot get on the floor. In these cases, therapy is often needed to help correct the condition.

When should my child start wearing shoes?

The barefoot baby is best as their muscles and feet discover how to adapt to surfaces. This helps to improve balance, coordination, and develop muscle strength. There is no need for a shoe until your child is walking, and then it is more for protection from the outside world. Flexible, soft shoes are the best choice for first shoes. No need to spend a lot of money on shoes for toddlers unless there is a medical issue and a special shoe is recommended by the pediatrician or podiatrist. It is best to find a good shoe store that is experienced in measuring feet, as it can be difficult to know the correct size. When in doubt go up in size to allow for growth.

What are growing pains?

Referring to the pain that some kids feel in their feet and legs as "growing pains" is one of my pet peeves. I personally do not give credence to this terminology. If growing hurt, every child would be in pain and that simply is not the case. When your child gets into bed at night and says "Mommy, my feet hurt" or "my legs hurt," this is really a cry for help.

In my experience, these children are often flat-footed or have feet that excessively pronate. This means their feet do not stay straight when they walk, and the inside of the feet, by the arch and ankle, falls inward. This falling in strains the muscles of the lower extremities, and when your child is active, the muscles fatigue more quickly. Hence, they get tired faster, and when finally done for the day, the muscles often spasm and ache. These pains are stress pains. They are usually easily corrected by simple arch supports or, as needed, specially designed inserts from your podiatrist. Kids who are placed into corrective orthotic inserts usually notice an immediate change and relief from fatiguing muscles and pain.

I first saw my patient Isabella, who is now five, just after she started walking. Although extremely bright and precocious, when she first came to the office, she was often irritable and refusing to walk. When I examined her, I found her feet totally collapsed inward. This explained her asking to be carried all the time. She was experiencing pain and fatigue due to stressed muscles. I fitted her for specialized custom orthotics to wear in her shoes that corrected the inward collapse. Within weeks she was walking, her spirits lifted, and she was no longer experiencing pain in her legs. Her parents report that she moves her orthotics from one pair of shoes to another all by herself. We replace her orthotics about every year and a half. Last time I saw Isabella, she told me, "I want my new orthotics!" She completely understands how they have changed her life.

My child doesn't like walking around the mall and often says "Mommy, carry me." What's wrong?

Remember Isabella's story above and understand these complaints are not usually signs of laziness. They are often signs of poorly functioning feet. If your child gets cranky and irritable when walking, please consider having their feet looked at.

Not all flat feet need treatment. There are normal flat feet and abnormal flat feet. It all depends on how they function. This again is something a quick specialty visit to the podiatrist can help you decipher. Is treatment needed or not? Find out. It can save your child years of foot fatigue and pain, and also secure a healthier adulthood for them.

Can children have the same foot problems as adults?

Throughout childhood, kids experience many of the same foot conditions as adults. In our practice we see children and teens with plantar warts, athlete's foot, ingrown toenails, heel pain, bunions, hammer toes, sprains, strains, and all kinds of injuries. Please use Part 2 of this book to answer questions you may have about any of these issues and to learn about possible treatment options for your child. As parents, let's remember the saying, "As the twig is bent, so grows the tree," and give our children sturdy roots and great healthy feet.

Chapter 4
The Fashionable Foot

To a podiatrist a healthy, pain-free, functioning foot is beautiful. Most foot owners, however, have different criteria. The foot has its power to attract, and throughout history people have been trying to enhance its charms. Queen Nefertiti painted her toenails—red, of course. Archeologists believe ancient Egyptians of both genders and all classes wore color on their nails and that the shade indicated their place in society, with the brightest used only by royalty. In thirteenth-century China, a small "lotus-shaped" foot was considered beautiful, and the feet of little girls were bound to curb their growth, often resulting in feet so deformed that walking was difficult. In some cultures, like northern Sumatra or Cambodia, large feet are thought most attractive because they are good for working in fields. Remember, beauty is in the eye of the beholder!

In our culture today, there are lots of options for adding foot appeal: softening, smoothing, painting nails, tattooing, wearing high heels, and yes, even cosmetic surgery. Some foot beautifying practices are harmless, but others can compromise foot health. In this chapter, I answer questions and offer tips about keeping your feet both beautiful and in good working order.

Pedicures

Pedicures have become wildly popular. Once the province of women, you now even hear pro football players mention their standing "pedi" appointments. I'm happy about this growing trend for both women and men to care for their feet, but I also have some dos and don'ts for making sure your feet stay healthy through the process, whether grooming at home or at the salon. Please note that diabetics are the exceptions to many of these rules and should seek professional advice.

Should I soak my feet?

Do soak your feet, but don't soak for too long. Feet work hard for us and deserve some spoiling now and then. I highly recommend soaking in Epsom salt, a combination of magnesium and sulfates. It feels good, soothes sore muscles, and your feet absorb the magnesium, which the body needs to regulate many critical functions. But be careful, soaking too long can dry out your skin and strip your feet of natural oils and minerals.

Should I trim down my calluses?

Trimming superficial calluses is fine, but don't take on deep or painful ones. As long as corns and calluses are not deep or painful and you are not diabetic or have poor circulation, go ahead and pumice or file down those areas with built-up skin. But stick to pumice stones or other friction-based callus removers, and avoid home or salon care that uses sharp instruments or blades. Always reserve work on deep bothersome corns and calluses for a podiatrist. Cuts or abrasions on the feet can lead to infection, so you only want an experienced professional to remove painful lesions. Foot doctors see patients with painful calluses all the time. It's part of our daily work, and we are happy to help you with them.

Is it okay to push back my cuticles?

I know showing more nail is considered more attractive, but this is a risky practice. Cuticles actually protect your nail. Being overaggressive in pushing them back or digging around or under the nails can cause microtrauma to the root, called the nail *matrix,* and affect nail growth. Microtrauma also can allow fungus to get a toehold. Podiatrists frequently see patients with problems after a pedicure. These patients may even confess that the pedicure was surprisingly painful when it was being done. If it hurts, chances are it isn't good for you!

Should I worry about the cleanliness of instruments at the nail salon?

Yes! Cleaning instruments with alcohol or cold sterilization techniques is often not good enough. Chances are those pedicure tools may still carry fungus and spores. Only very high temperatures can guarantee sterilization and killing of all disease-causing germs. That's why medical offices and operating rooms have autoclaves that heat instruments to temperatures high enough to kill all fungi, spores, and bacteria. Salons don't autoclave, which is why fungal infections can be spread so easily among customers. I recommend purchasing your own pedicure kit, bringing it with you to the salon, and asking the pedicurist to use only your personal instruments on your feet. Don't feel awkward. This is an increasingly common practice.

Should the pedicurist tackle my ingrown toenail?

Unfortunately, I see far too many patients with infections caused by untrained people attempting to remove an ingrown nail border, either at home or at the nail salon. Do see a podiatrist to treat the nail. Don't suffer—have it taken care of by an experienced foot doctor. (See Chapter 8 for more about treatment of ingrown nails.)

Is it healthy to wear nail polish?

Don't wear polish all the time. Give your nails a chance to breathe. Polish seals nails off from oxygen, creating an inviting environment for fungus and bacteria to set up shop. When the summer sandal-wearing season is over, we always see women in our offices who have removed nail polish after wearing it for several months, only to be horrified to see a nail is no longer a healthy pink color. It has become discolored by a new shade of white, yellow, or grey—the result of a fungus invasion. Chapter 7 offers both home remedies and podiatrist protocols for toenail fungus, which can be extremely difficult to get rid of.

Do seek out nontoxic polishes. Modern nail polish is essentially paint and contains many toxic ingredients including formaldehyde, toluene, and preservatives. These toxins are damaging to the body and can be absorbed through the skin, nails, and lungs. New York City now has strict laws governing the air quality of nail salons to protect people from breathing in these harmful chemicals. I recommend nontoxic polishes, which are free of unhealthy chemicals. Many of these polishes also allow oxygen to pass through, and some contain antifungal agents. We offer nontoxic nail polishes at our offices, and you can also find them on our website, *askthefootdoctor.com.*

Are foot massages good for your feet?

A foot massage feels terrific and is a great stress reliever. Your feet have many muscles and nerve endings that benefit from massage, and they surely deserve the attention. Find a friend or family member and trade foot massages— your feet will thank you.

Tattooing

No doctors advocate tattoos, but many people find them a fun form of self-expression. My recommendation, if you are considering a foot tattoo, is to avoid the sides of the ankle. This area has thin skin and many nerves. In fact, I would avoid the foot altogether and opt for the leg above the ankle for a tattoo site.

High Heels

Fortunately for me, heels have been out of fashion for standard male wear for centuries. Historians think heels were first worn by Persian horsemen to keep their feet from slipping out of stirrups—a reasonable functional enhancement. Today they are worn to give the foot a graceful arch and show off a shapely leg. High heels may be considered sexy, but I don't need to tell you that walking on the balls of your feet is neither efficient nor comfortable.

The design of women's dress shoes places the foot at an angle that aggravates or, in some cases, causes foot problems including bunions, neuromas (pinched nerves), hammer toes, *metatarsalgia* (painful metatarsals—the long bones in the feet), and much more. What you do every once in a while may not be harmful; however, a frequent wearer of high heels is much more likely to require the services of a skilled podiatrist sooner or later. Although high heels are not the cause of all foot problems, they certainly are the cause of many painful feet.

Does anyone make comfortable high heels?

Most shoe designers are male and this may explain why so little thought is put into a woman's comfort while wearing shoes. There are new designs that do attempt to balance style and function. Here are some tips to keep in mind when choosing heels. Opt for a thicker heel as opposed to a stiletto. The thicker heel allows for less wobble and more stability and distributes the weight more evenly under the heel. A platform also is better than a thin sole because a thin sole puts excessive pressure on the ball of the foot. Adding a silicone pad under the ball of the foot may help too. Lastly, if you must wear high heels, limit the time you spend in them, make sure you avoid shoes that cause your feet to hurt, and stretch your leg muscles and calf areas so the muscles and tendons don't shorten from prolonged wear.

Cosmetic Foot Surgery

The narrow pointy toe areas of most high heels and fashion shoes confine and constrict feet. Nowadays it is not uncommon for a woman to request surgery to reshape her feet for a better fit in these shoes. I don't perform or recommend this kind of cosmetic surgery. When considering any surgery, you must always ask, "Are the rewards worth the risk?" My best advice is to reward yourself and your feet with comfortable shoes.

Some women inquire about foot surgery to improve the look of their foot. "Slimming" toes to appear less chunky or shortening a longer toe are surgeries performed in some cities where designer shoes are de rigueur. Foot surgery is usually not recommended unless it relieves a painful problem or improves the function of a patient's foot. Ideal or perfect feet should not be our goal! Besides, the ideal is relative. It changes with different cultures and different historical periods. Feet that get you where you want to go without complaint are what truly stand the test of time.

Chapter 5

Fun and Games:
Prevent, Prepare, and Play Like a Pro

Every day I look forward to my run. Whether I'm at home or traveling, whether I run along roads or on my favorite trail, across a city or up a lonely mountain, whether I'm with my running partner or by myself or packed beside thousands at the start of a race, my run energizes me. Running has been my primary source of exercise for most of my adult life and has brought me joy, a healthy lifestyle, and community. Running inspires me and is one of the reasons I chose to become a podiatrist. I enjoy being around other runners and athletes and helping them achieve their goals. I also encourage all my patients to become fitness focused and discover the benefits of exercise.

Over the years, I have treated many patients with running and sports injuries who seek out our office to get "back on their feet." I have found that every level of athlete, from the committed to the weekend warrior, from the beginner to the expert, is vulnerable to foot problems. An injured foot can not only take you out of the game, it can lay you up, keeping you from play and work. Some foot injuries are unavoidable, but others you can steer clear of if you take some basic precautions.

Prepare Like a Pro

The first step in avoiding injury is to be prepared. Think spring training. Baseball players show up at camp after months off to prepare their bodies for the demands ahead. A professional athlete would never jump into a season without properly training beforehand. And you and I shouldn't either. I'm still waiting for my patient Robert to learn that lesson. Robert is a forty-four-year-old weekend warrior who loves softball. His day job is at a desk, and every year when the weather warms up in the Northeast, he dons his baseball glove and heads out to the diamond. It never fails, each year he arrives at the office with another injury, Achilles tendonitis, plantar fasciitis, stress fracture, to name just a few. He grins and says he must be getting old. Each year I tell him the same thing: "You can't just go out and play like you're a teenager. You have to get into shape first."

Our bodies are in shape to do what we have been doing. Been cycling every other day? Your body is used to it. Been walking six blocks from the train station to the office Monday through Friday? Your body's got you covered. Been watching ESPN from your couch every weekend? Your system is perfectly tuned for it. But add a new demand, and your body will feel it—stress. Any change in our routine activity level stresses the body and makes it vulnerable to injury.

It is important to understand stress is a relative term. This means that stress is different for every person. What the body perceives as stress is based on what that particular body is accustomed to doing on a daily basis.

For athletes, stress injuries are caused by rapidly increasing intensity, speed, mileage, weights, or duration of workouts. Changing from one sport to another is also stressful. Each sport requires muscles to function differently. A runner who logs five miles daily easily develops sore muscles and strained tendons by going out and playing basketball, if basketball is not part of his or her regular routine.

The rule is, if the activity is new or you are taking it to a new level, take it slowly. I recommend this for people at all fitness levels. Carefully plan your entry. Don't go whole hog; devise a program that gradually progresses to where you want to be. Slow and steady means you lower the chances of being laid up by an injury. Slow and steady means you'll be able to meet your goals—a race, a weekly league, or shooting hoops and trying to keep up with the kids.

Warm Up Like a Pro

A gradual buildup to a season or new activity is preparing for the long term, but you should also have a routine to prep your body before you take off down the trail or the whistle blows to start the game. Warming up is a must and includes stretching. Again, we should take a lesson from the professionals. We see pro athletes warming up all the time, and what we see them doing on the field or court is just the end of a routine that started in the locker room, or even when they first got out of bed in the morning.

Should I stretch before exercise?

Yes, stretch as much as you can! This includes the feet and the leg muscles too. With 26 bones, 19 muscles, 109 ligaments, 33 joints, and 42 tendons, there's a lot in a foot that can go wrong. It would be great if the body came with a warning sign: "Avoid cold starts. Warm up your engine before heavy use."

I am a huge advocate of stretching and transforming your body slowly over time. Daily stretching is a vital component to sustain tip-top shape for a lifetime. The most important muscles to stretch in addition to your feet include your calf muscles, your hamstrings, and your lower back. There are so many different theories on stretching, and the literature continues to be rife with varying opinions. My preferred stretching techniques are short three-second stretches of each muscle group, repeating reps of ten. In the past, longer sustained stretching was usually preferred; however, the shorter stretches repeated multiple times have proven to be a better choice for warming up and getting ready for action.

Stretching takes time. Don't rush. Each day may seem like a struggle, but, the long-term benefits are worth it. To view the recommended stretches for each important muscle group, please visit our website at *askthefootdoctor.com for a how-to visual tutorial.*

Do I need a different pair of shoes for every sport I play?

Short answer—yes. Shoes play an important role in protecting your foot function, so make sure you wear the right ones for the activity. Different sports stress our feet in different ways. Sport-specific shoes are designed to help your feet meet the particular demands of your sport. Tennis shoes are designed for quick starts and stops and side-to-side support. There are even different tennis shoes for different surfaces. Basketball shoes provide traction, support, and durability. Soccer players require shoes or cleats that match the various surfaces they play on, while maintaining support and helping add power and control for kicking the ball. Runners need the right shoe for their particular foot. This may be a shoe that offers motion control and support, or a style that blends maximal cushioning for shock absorption. The right shoes will go a long way in helping guard against injury. They are worth the investment. For more about choosing running shoes, a favorite topic of the running podiatrist, visit our website at *askthefootdoctor.com.*

How can I avoid ankle injury?

It is almost unheard of for professional athletes to compete in certain sports without getting their ankles taped up before competition. This simple preventive measure averts many ankle injuries. Once an ankle has been sprained a number of times, the ligaments are stretched out and can't properly do their job of holding the ankle bones firmly in place, which makes the ankle more likely to be sprained yet again.

We may not have our spouses tape us up before we attack our nine-to-five jobs, but it is a consideration before we become weekend warriors. In addition to using sports tape, off-the-shelf ankle braces are readily available to help support and protect your ankles. If you have prior history of ankle injury, taping or bracing is a must. Chapter 15 offers more about ankle injury prevention and treatment.

When should I get my injured foot checked out?

Swelling, pain, and difficulty walking are immediate signs that you need to seek professional evaluation. Often if our feet or ankles hurt, we just keep going, hoping they will get better. The danger is the longer we go without treatment, the harder some injuries are to heal. An x-ray quickly reveals whether or not you have broken bones, but that x-ray does not show damage to ligaments or tendons. Just getting the "all clear" that there is no break does not mean you are out of the woods.

There is a saying that a sprain can be worse than a break. This is because a broken bone is diagnosed and treated quickly, while a ligament injury often goes undiagnosed. Ligaments may often need rehabilitation and sometimes repair. Let a podiatrist determine if you need treatment and explore the options with you. If you are having particular trouble with your ankle, check out Chapter 15, and if your Achilles tendon is tender, see Chapter 14.

How do I avoid getting blisters?

Most athletes and runners don't get blisters, thank goodness, but those that do seem to get them frequently. Usual blister areas include the toes, heels, or bottoms of the feet. A blister begins as a hot spot that may get red and uncomfortable. If the culprit—friction—continues, a full-fledged fluid-filled blister forms.

There are three principal causes of blister-inducing friction on the foot. A too snug shoe is the most common. When buying shoes, keep in mind that the best fit usually has about a thumbnail's width of room between your toes and the end of the shoe. Your socks can also be giving you the wrong rub. Again a good comfortable fit is important to avoid friction, but don't overlook the sock material. Cotton is not best for sports socks. Although cotton absorbs moisture, it also retains it so the sweat is left in contact with the skin, which can lead to blisters. Most runners and athletes wear socks made of synthetic materials that "wick" moisture away from the skin. A simple change from cotton to synthetic "blister-free" socks can reduce blister formation significantly. And there's always Vaseline. At a marathon the jars fly as runners slather petroleum jelly on every potential blister area.

Should I pop or not?

If the blister is not painful and you have time to let it heal, it can take care of itself. If you have pain, need to run, play, or workout and your blister is filled with fluid, it is best to drain it. Sterilize a small needle and pop the blister in one or two areas. Do not "de-roof" the blister. Leave the soft blister skin intact after draining the fluid. If you peel the skin off, it usually creates even more pain. Cover it with antiseptic and a Band-Aid until healed.

It is possible for a blister to get infected, although not common. If there is any excessive redness, pain, or discharge from the area, visit your podiatrist. Our office gets especially busy before and after marathons with patients who have painful blisters and need professional attention to relieve pain quickly.

What if I'm an athlete with foot symptoms not mentioned here?

There are many foot conditions that athletes frequently contend with. See Part 2 of this book to get the rundown on other common foot problems like heel pain, tendonitis, stress fractures, broken toes, sprained ankles, ingrown nails, athlete's foot, fungus, and more. Don't suffer, get informed, seek treatment, and prevent, prepare, and play like a pro.

Chapter 6

Seniors:
Feet Don't Fail Me Now

---

have been a practicing foot doctor for over thirty years. That means I've had long relationships with many of my patients. I've treated children who are now grown and bring their own children to see me. I've first treated patients in their fifties and cared for them into their eighties. And I have some patients I started seeing when they were in their seventies who are now more than a hundred years old. I've watched many pairs of feet age. In fact, about 25 percent of my patients are over sixty-five. From them I have learned what is valued and vital for a rewarding senior life—staying active and independent.

Sir Isaac Newton put forward the laws of motion several centuries ago. One of the laws is that an object that is in motion tends to stay in motion. In our golden years, we want to be able to dance with our spouse, take walks with our grandkids, stroll along the beach with a friend. Making those dreams come true depends on our health and especially our feet. Even being able to care for our homes and ourselves depends so much on mobility. Our very independence is linked to feet that can get us around. And there is no question that Newton's law applies to seniors: the more active we are, the more active we continue to be.

I can't deny physical changes are inevitable as we age. Our eyes, our teeth, our hair, our skin all change with time. And our feet change too, just like the rest of us. The shape of our feet, our toenails, the skin on our feet, the density of our bones, can dramatically alter as we enter our senior years. How our feet feel changes as well. Feet may start to tire quickly and develop more aches and pains. The good news is, although we have no remedy yet for aging, there are choices we can make to keep us moving and enjoying life's pleasures.

Let's take a look at some of the changes that most of us experience to some degree as we climb in years and their consequences for our feet. Then we'll talk about what you can do to keep you and your feet in motion.

Bone Density

Our bones can lose density as we grow older. This causes them to become weaker and brittle and more vulnerable to fractures. Age, heredity, and gender are all factors in developing *osteoporosis,* or bone loss. Women are affected more than men. Osteoporosis also tends to run in families. Though bone loss can occur at any age, most people start to lose bone density in their fifties. Over ten million women in the US are said to have osteoporosis, with another thirty-four million having osteopenia, which is lower than normal bone mass and a precursor to osteoporosis.

If I have osteoporosis are my feet affected?

Though you most often hear of seniors having hip fractures due to weakened bones, senior feet are vulnerable to fractures as well. Stress fractures are hairline fractures that commonly occur in the long metatarsal bones of the foot. Beware: Pain and swelling on top of the foot could indicate a possible stress fracture. See a podiatrist for an x-ray to make sure you are not walking on a broken bone. Immediate treatment is necessary to ensure bone healing.

If diagnosed with osteoporosis, supportive shoes with extra cushioning are a must. Also, limit excessive activities and be careful not to overdo it on vacations. Avoid walking barefoot, even in the house, to protect your feet. Advancing osteoporosis makes it more difficult for your feet to carry your body around like it used to. Proper nutrition is a must to ensure your body is getting what it needs to stay healthy. With osteoporosis, it is difficult to play catch up and modern medicine has no cure yet. Keeping active is the best medicine and also the better way to beat back the advances of bone loss.

Muscle Power

Muscles create power and motion, but they naturally weaken as we age. Decreased muscle mass means less strength and declining mobility. Heredity, hormonal changes, lack of exercise, diet, and illness all contribute to muscles becoming weaker. Unfortunately, too many seniors ignore their muscles and the importance of keeping muscles strong and toned.

What happens to my feet if they lose muscle strength?

Feet are especially susceptible to loss of muscle strength and function. There are over one hundred muscles, tendons, and ligaments in each foot. These help us walk and give support and stability to our body. When foot muscles and tendons lose even a portion of their strength, feet often begin to change. The saying, "if you don't use it, you lose it," applies to your muscles and to bone density. Exercise helps to keep your muscles and bones strong, along with aiding your circulation and cardiac fitness.

Changes due to loss of foot strength can occur slowly and take different forms. For some, the feet become flatter and the arch disappears. For others feet begin to look different as toes change shape and position. Hammer toes and bunions may grow faster. Feet may become tired more quickly, forcing more frequent rest and reducing desire to be active. Some people may begin to feel less stable on their feet and fear losing their balance. For many seniors, there is just more foot pain than there used to be. What used to be done with ease is no longer a breeze.

Joints and Arthritis

The more birthdays we have, the greater the chance of developing arthritis that slows us down and limits our mobility. Arthritis affects our bones and joints. Injuries, systemic conditions, and just plain wear and tear cause an increased likelihood of joint pain as we age. Injuries or accidents throughout our lifetime can be exacerbated and years later develop into arthritis.

Can I have arthritis in my feet?

Many people experience arthritis in the joints of their feet. Any joint in the body can develop arthritis, and because the feet have so many joints, thirty-three to be exact, the chances of developing arthritis in your feet is significant. The big toe joint is especially susceptible. There are options for treatment depending on the type of arthritis and which joint is affected. But remember that unlike a hip or knee—a single large joint that can be replaced—the foot's joints are many and work in a complex harmony. Foot joint replacements are rarely the best option. Arthritis and treatments are discussed in much greater detail in Chapter 17.

Taking Action

You can build muscle and bone strength and keep joints limber to enhance the mobility of your senior years. Muscles, bones, and joints all respond to being worked. They respond to exercise. I want to say this loudly: **You are never too old to start exercising and to reap the benefits. I have many patients who have made changes in their exercise habits in their senior years and experienced great improvement in their quality of life. Walking, swimming, taking an aqua-aerobics class, biking, participating in Pilates or yoga, stretching—these are all activities that build strength and flexibility and are ingredients for happy senior living. Find a gym or senior exercise class in your community. It feels great to be active and participating. To get you started, I've outlined the benefits of some activities below and included a couple more options for improving your foot health. Choose one or several from the list and just do it!**

Walk

Study after study shows the benefits of a walking program to maintain health and fitness. A brisk walk that elevates your heart rate is best; however, any walking, even a stroll, has benefits. Your feet want you to see the world, so take a walk every day. Go on your own or find a walking partner. Take a walking class at the YMCA or your local recreation department. I taught a class in how to start a walking program at a local community college. It was so rewarding to help seniors get started on their journey to better health. Simple walking is free, easy, and has major benefits. No excuses, just lace up your shoes, get out the door, and start putting one foot in front of the other!

Keep Your Muscles Strong

There are many ways to build muscle and strength. Exercising with weights is one of them. You don't need to use heavy weights. There is a risk of injury if the weights are too heavy. It is best to use lighter weights or elastic bands and do more repetitions. Practice toe raises to keep your feet strong. Start with two feet and advance to one foot if you can. Progress to balance exercises by standing on one foot, holding onto something as needed to prevent falling. Do not struggle; be comfortable. Consider a personal trainer. A trainer keeps you motivated and ensures your form is correct, minimizing injury risk.

Stretch

The classic mental image of an elderly person is of a stooped, frail figure clutching a cane or walker, their feet shuffling in short little steps as they barely move along. This senior's gait is stiff and inflexible because of tight joints and muscles that no longer have any elasticity. Can this shuffling scenario be avoided? For many, a regular routine of stretching exercises helps.

If there is one thing I recommend more than anything else to keep mobile in your senior years, it is stretching. If you work to keep yourself flexible, your stride may not shorten much as you age. Join a stretching class at a local gym. A yoga program or Pilate's classes are also good choices. A class designed specifically for seniors is your best bet. Stretching is like brushing your teeth—it should be done daily. Develop your own program. Stick to it, and remember it's never too late to start stretching. One day, your ninety-year-old you will thank you.

Take an Aqua-Aerobics Class

Find a gym with a pool that offers water classes. Water aerobics is a great form of exercise. Music, a fun instructor, and the company of others, make this a perfect way to stay fit. It is also easier on painful feet.

Bicycle

Riding a stationary bicycle or an outdoor bicycle is also great exercise, especially for those with painful feet or knees. It doesn't take long to get some daily exercise in, and for many this is an excellent choice to keep body parts in motion.

Lose Those Extra Pounds

Excessive body weight is hard on your feet. They are forced to carry the burden each and every step. If you pack an extra 30 to 50 pounds, this can cause tremendous foot pain over time. Being overweight flattens feet, causes tendon strain, heel spurs, arch pain, chronic fatigue, and generalized foot pain. It also strains the heart and many other critical body functions. One of the quickest ways to get old fast is to gain weight. I often recommend that my overweight patients, senior or not, see a nutritionist and start making healthy diet choices. Those who do, find their feet feel the difference.

Wear Good Shoes

Comfort, cushioning, support, and stability are the keys to the best shoes for seniors. Who cares what they look like? Remember, fashion is for kids. Comfort is for the experienced. Review the four tests for "good" shoes in Chapter 2.

Don't Be a Homebody

It's better to be a busy body. Keep your body busy. Get out and do things. Walk in the local charity events. Volunteer. Join a gym. Go on a senior trip. Garden. Take a class at the local college. Keep your brain and mind stimulated too. Play word games, memory games, and read stimulating books and magazines. Visit the library. Keep active. Have a daily plan. Make sure there is something you enjoy and look forward to on your calendar every day—something to keep you moving.

Taking Care of "Small" Foot Issues

Besides the "biggies"—bone loss, muscle loss, and arthritis—seniors do face some smaller but often very limiting foot problems: thick fungus nails, painful corns and calluses, dropped metatarsals, thinning of the skin on the bottom of the feet, to name a few. Make no mistake, these "minor" foot issues can stop you in your tracks and keep you from moving and reaping all the physical and psychological benefits of being active. My advice is to be like the patients in the stories I share below and seek routine help from your foot doctor with both "lesser" and greater foot problems alike.

Senior Success Stories

Carl was a reluctant patient when he first came to see me some twenty years ago. He didn't think his foot pain really warranted a doctor's visit, and he did not like to admit that he couldn't manage his own foot care anymore. Carl had deep painful calluses on the bottoms of his feet that formed because his metatarsal bones had dropped. His toenails had also thickened and curved and overgrew so badly they hampered his walking.

Though Carl's problems were not "curable," I have helped him maintain and enjoy a good quality of life. I see Carl every third Tuesday of every other month, and provide enough relief for him to keep up his daily visits to the YMCA. At the Y, he walks a treadmill for several miles then goes to the exercise room for light weight work and stretching. Because Carl took action about his feet, he has been able to stay in motion, and his daily exercise routine is the key to his also staying able and young at heart.

Sally Ann is another longtime patient. She has arthritis, hammer toes, calluses, and terrible toenails. Regular podiatric appointments have enabled her to keep walking, playing the organ, and visiting senior homes to share music with the residents. Her foot care routine has added quality to her life and to those she entertains, as well as allowing her to enjoy time with her husband, Michael.

As you or someone you care for begins to experience foot changes, I hope you will remember staying in motion is essential. Make a podiatrist your new best friend. Don't give up on your dreams for your golden years. Make the choices that will keep you on your feet and independent.

Part 2

———

Your Foot and Ankle:

Conditions, Causes, and Cures

"Can I Ask You a Question?"
A Guide to Part 2

"Hey Doc, can I ask you something?" It never fails—whenever someone finds out I'm a podiatrist, I get asked that question. At parties, on planes, in restaurants, at sporting events, even at the movies, people sidle up, give me a nudge, and ask if they can ask. And as soon as I say, "Sure, ask away," a shoe slips off and the questions just keep on coming.

If you have questions about your feet, you are not alone. Everyone does! There are so many little things that can be a bother, and so many bigger things that can be a real pain. Getting simple questions answered is a service I am glad to provide anytime. It always feels good to take the worry, fear, or pain away and start someone off on the path to resolving his or her foot complaint, however minor or major it may be.

When I see patients in the office, I have the same goal and policy. I want my patients to ask about whatever is bothering them. During their exam, diagnosis, and treatment explanation, I want them to ask me questions until they fully understand what caused the foot issue, what they can do to make the problem better, and what I can do to help them.

Part 2 of this book is designed to be your chance to consult the foot doctor. You say, "Doctor Tumen, you got a minute?" And I say, "You bet." You slip your shoe off, and we'll take a look together. You get to ask as many questions as

41

you want. And I explain as thoroughly as I can and give you as many treatment options as I think helpful, including home care, for dealing with your foot condition.

Each chapter in this part of the book covers a specific foot problem. I start the chapters by giving you a good idea of what the condition looks like and feels like. From there the chapters follow a question-and-answer format about causes, home treatment, when you should go to a doctor, what the doctor is going to do to diagnose your foot challenge, and what the doctor can do to relieve your pain and fix the problem.

I've focused on the foot problems we see most often in our practice. They fall into four main categories. Soft tissue issues are first up with chapters on fungus toenails, plantar warts, and ingrown toenails. Though not the most serious of foot conditions, soft tissue problems can be vexing, painful, and worst of all, recurring or spreading.

Next are the bunion and hammer toe chapters, which fall under deformities (such a scary word for a wonky toe or two). These usually develop slowly over time or are a foot trait inherited from Mom or Dad or Grandma. Thanks, Grandma! Bunions and hammer toes can become painful and hamper walking.

The third batch of chapters is the largest and covers foot problems that are caused by injury or overuse. These include Morton's neuroma, which is a pinched nerve in the ball of the foot; plantar fasciitis, which typically gives the sufferer a pain in the heel; Achilles tendon troubles; broken toes (please, pay attention to these); and ankle injuries, with a detailed discussion of sprains.

Last but not least are the chapters dealing with foot problems that may be the result of larger overall health or systemic issues: arthritis, diabetes, and gout. In addition to focusing on how these conditions affect the feet, I broaden the discussion to help you understand these larger health challenges. I also give recommendations for changes you can make that might help you better manage these conditions and improve your health in general.

After you find and read the chapter that matches your foot problem, I hope you feel educated about the condition and ready to tackle it. That's the first step to solving a foot issue. The next step is to make an appointment with a podiatrist. Why do you need to see a podiatrist if you are going to get such complete information from *Ask the Foot Doctor?* Three reasons:

1. *Feet shouldn't hurt,* and you shouldn't continue to suffer with a foot problem. While some foot conditions may improve on their own or with home care, the majority require professional evaluation and a treatment plan to heal or to prevent the issue from continuing to worsen, recur, or develop into a complication.

2. *Many foot problems overlap.* One condition may cause or be a by-product of another. A podiatrist can evaluate the big picture, diagnose the foot as a whole rather than individual parts, and often solve longstanding or recurring issues.

3. *No two feet are exactly alike*—even the two in a pair are different. That means in order to have your feet evaluated accurately, you will have to trot them in to a foot doctor.

How do I choose a podiatrist?

Look for a podiatrist who is board certified or board qualified. This indicates he or she has met stringent qualifications and the highest standards of the profession. Podiatrists usually have these certifications listed on their website and often after their names on their cards.

A good reputation is important so start by asking around. Get a suggestion from your primary care physician, ask other health professionals that you know, get a recommendation from friends.

Professional and helpful staff is a good indicator of a caring practice with high standards. Take note when you are making an appointment or arriving at the office—is the staff cheerful, friendly, and efficient? Also check out waiting rooms and examining rooms. They should be clean and up-to-date.

Your podiatrist should be thorough. During the exam, your podiatrist should ask you about your medical history, listen to your symptoms, and take the time to examine every part of your foot.

Your podiatrist should give clear explanations of your condition and your treatment options, and of course, answer all questions. Ask yourself if you understood the diagnosis you were given and the plan of action for resolving your foot issue. Do you know what the next step is? Do you know what you should or should not be doing at home?

Trust your gut. Does your podiatrist listen to you? Do you feel that he or she has your best interests at heart? You know the feeling you get when you are seen by your doctor. If it's a feeling of trust, trust it. If it isn't, move on to another foot specialist.

In order to understand your feet, podiatrists have to know a lot about you: what your job is, what activities you participate in, what you enjoy doing, what your goals are. Your podiatrist is also probably going to be seeing you over time. Many foot issues require careful follow-up, so podiatrists tend to be more involved with patients and develop long-term connections with their patients and families. In short, you are going to have a real relationship with your foot doctor. So choose someone you are comfortable with, who is knowledgeable, confident, encouraging, and who wants you to enjoy your life to the fullest. You and your feet deserve that!

Before we move on, I want to say a few words about surgery. No need to start worrying, the majority of foot issues do not require surgery, but sometimes surgery is necessary and important. You will see that in each chapter in Part 2, I tell you if surgery is a treatment option and when it may be time to consider it. If surgery is an option you are weighing, please consult Chapter 20 at the end of Part 2. In that chapter, I discuss how to choose a surgeon, what questions to ask, and what to think about before scheduling a procedure. You call the shots when it comes to surgery, and I want you to have the information you need to get the best result for you and your feet.

Now, slip off your shoes and socks, put your feet up, and let's walk through the rest of the book together. It's time to turn the page on foot problems.

Chapter 7

Fungus Nails:
There's No Fun in Fungus

I f you have a fungus nail, you are not alone! Forty-three million Americans, about 14 percent of the population, have this condition, medically known as *onychomycosis*. The first sign usually is gradual discoloration of one or more nails. They may turn various shades of yellow, gray, black, or white. The nail also thickens, can be near impossible to cut, and may even become painful. The fungus can spread from one toenail to two to all and prove stubborn to cure. You can fight the fungus invasion and even win, many of my patients do, but it takes patience and . . . a little bit of luck.

Who can get a fungus nail?

Anyone can get a fungus toenail. Fungus is always among us, awaiting opportunity. A recent study reported (believe it or not) that about two hundred different species of fungi exist on the feet alone. In a sampling of toenail clippings from just ten people, over sixty different species of fungus were isolated!

Why is there so much fungus on feet?

Think about the living conditions of our feet. They are encapsulated in shoes for an average of eight to fourteen hours a day. The inside of a shoe is a dark place without much air circulation, and before putting our feet in the shoe, we also wrap them in socks that block air. Nylon stockings in particular don't breathe well, suffocating the feet. Our feet also add moisture to their environment, sweating more than we might know or would ever admit. The average foot has approximately 250,000 sweat glands, and feet sweat on average about a half pint a day.

In addition, the average person takes thousands of steps per day, sometimes in shoes that may be a tad uncomfortable. This creates microtrauma to the feet, with the toes often bearing the brunt. Microtrauma is not painful like getting your toe stepped on. It is repetitive stress, similar to typing on a keyboard and developing carpal tunnel syndrome in the wrist.

So, combine darkness with no air circulation between the toes, add a dash of moisture, mix in a modest amount of microtrauma, and you have the perfect recipe for fungus to thrive and stay alive.

The Good Guys versus the Bad Guys

It is important to know there are good fungi and not-so-good fungi. Think about penicillin, which is made from a fungus. That's a good one. Then there is the fungus *Trichophyton rubrum (T. rubrum)*, which is the fungus most commonly responsible for fungus toenails. This bad guy is not your favorite fungus. There is a constant battle waging between the good and the bad fungi on your feet, and sometimes the bad guys win and take over the real estate of your toenail.

Why the nail?

Fungi do not make their own food; they need a source. Hence, the toenail becomes the source. Fungus can remain in just a part of one toenail, or eventually it can spread into all ten toenails.

Can the fungus spread to other parts of the body?

Like Las Vegas, what happens in the toenails usually stays in the toenails, although on occasion it is possible to spread from the nails to the adjoining skin.

Can I give the fungus to my spouse?

In my experience, I do not see a strong tendency to contract a fungus toenail from a partner. Although it is possible, it is not common. So feel free to play footsie and not worry so much. However, if your partner has athlete's foot, take care because that is more contagious (see Athlete's Foot section below).

Why did my feet lose the battle against the bad foot fungi?

As in any war, there are any number of circumstances and events that can turn the tide. Let's take a look at some of the most common causes for good fungi losing ground to the bad fungi on your feet.

Trauma

An injury to the toe can disrupt the balance between the good and the bad fungi, allowing the bad fungus to begin its takeover of the nail. Frozen food falling from the freezer and scoring a direct hit on the toe has caused many fungus toenails. Banging toes into chairs and walls also is a common cause of damaged nails and fungus invasion.

Sports Injuries

Although sports injuries fall into the trauma category, runners and other athletes develop toenail fungus at higher rates than the average population. This is often because of both direct trauma and microtrauma. In my practice, distance runners often display their deformed toenails like a badge of courage. A great marathon story complete with bloody socks and lost toenails usually accompanies the runner with "ugly toenail syndrome."

Athlete's Foot

Often found between toes and on the bottom of the feet, athlete's foot, known as *tinea pedis,* is caused by fungi. If athlete's foot is present, there is a greater chance of fungus finding a way to invade your toenails. It is important to know that athlete's foot is easy to get and commonly spread around locker rooms, gyms, and showers. So if there is a spouse in the house who has athlete's foot, get it treated so it is not a cause of fungus taking up residence on your foot or toenails.

Ingrown Toenail

Although we focus on ingrown toenails in Chapter 8, it is important to mention that chronic ingrown nails can also be a factor in developing fungus toenails.

Shoes

It is worth saying again that uncomfortable shoes may contribute to fungus toenails. This caution is especially important for women who wear dress shoes. Squeezing your feet on a regular basis into Manolo Blahnik's and other dress shoes that do not have enough room for your toes is a no-no for many reasons. The daily repetitive trauma to the toes damages the integrity of the nails and allows for fungus to set up shop. It's best to buy comfy shoes with lots of (or at least a little more) room in the toe box, so your toes can wiggle at will.

Nail Polish

In Chapter 4, "The Fashionable Foot," I discuss nail polish in detail, but here are the basics. Polishes cut off the nail from oxygen and have toxic ingredients that create an environment that fungi actually find inviting. The longer the polish is worn, the more likely a fungus is to make the nail a home, often going undetected under the polish. I am not against nail polish, I just advocate making good polish choices. See our website at *askthefootdoctor.com* for recommendations for newer and healthier toenail polishes that have removed all toxins and also include antifungal ingredients.

Pedicures

Although it's unlikely you will give your partner toenail fungus, it is not uncommon to pick up someone else's bad fungus at the nail salon. Why? Although instruments are always cleaned between customers, some strains of fungus can be difficult to eradicate and are spread from one customer to another. I recommend purchasing your own grooming kit and asking your nail technician to use your personal instruments on your feet. In addition (yes, there is more,) digging under the cuticles and under the nails, and pushing the skin back from the nail can cause trauma, opening the door for bad fungus. For more dos and don'ts of pedicures and foot beautifying practices see Chapter 4, "The Fashionable Foot."

Heredity

Unfortunately, you can do everything right and still end up with fungus toenails. Fungus, like many other conditions tends to run in families. We do sometimes become our mothers and fathers. So if Dad had fungus toenails, you may end up with them too.

Age

The age-old question, is age a factor? And the answer is yes. Healthy, pretty toenails are the property of the young. Wrinkles, grey hair, and fungus toenails belong to the experienced. If you are in the over sixty club, about 60 percent of this population has fungus in one or more toenails. Of course, all the other factors listed here can also play into the development of fungus toenails in seniors.

Diabetes

Diabetes causes many foot problems, and diabetics have a higher percentage of toenail fungus than the general population.

Circulation

Poor circulation can be a by-product of age, diabetes, or other health issues. Keep in mind that the weaker your circulation, the greater your chance of developing fungus toenails. Good blood supply and oxygen circulating in full force to the tips of your toes help keep toenails healthy.

Other Systemic Conditions

To be thorough, I must mention that there are many additional health challenges that can cause toenails to change color and thicken. Psoriasis, arthritis, lung diseases, and chemotherapy are just a few. Remember that we are one body from top to bottom, so in general, the healthier your body, the healthier your toenails.

How do I get rid of a fungus toenail?

Not all fungus toenails can be cured. That is a hard thing to hear if you are one of the millions sprouting a fungus toenail and wanting to know the latest and greatest miracle treatment. Miracles may be around the corner, they are just not here yet.

Of course, I have heard many a patient say, "Doc, we can send a man to the moon, but you can't cure my toenail fungus?" No argument here. We are working on it and although we can't win all fungus battles, we can win many.

My recommendation is at the first sign of discoloration or thickening of a nail, seek a podiatrist for evaluation and treatment. It's much easier to treat a fungus toenail when first spotted. It becomes more challenging when the nail becomes thickened and multiple nails are involved. That said, I know if you seek advice from friends or on the Internet, you will come across many home remedies, so I want to talk about some of those here. Then I'll discuss using topical antifungal agents, and finally present treatment options your podiatrist can offer.

What are some home remedies for toenail fungus?

Often when there are many remedies, it is because none works very well. Most home treatments have a fairly low cure rate, usually less than 10 percent, and those cures are almost always for simple early-onset cases. When any home remedy is successful, it is due to patience, consistency, and luck. Here are a few podiatric tips for dealing with a fungus toenail at home. Make sure you trim the affected nail as low as possible to physically remove as much of the bad nail as you can. Do not lift the nail off the nail bed, and don't attempt to dig under the nail. Digging under the nail may separate the nail from the underlying nail bed, making it easier for fungus to thrive.

Let it be known that the following home "cures" are not recommendations, but are included to be complete in our discussion.

Vicks VapoRub

Of all the home remedies, Vicks VapoRub appears to be the most popular. Many with a fungus toenail have found the Vicks in the medicine cabinet and started dabbing it on a toenail or two. Why would it work? Most likely it's because Vicks contains an ingredient called thymol, which is a thyme derivative. Thymol oil or thyme has been shown to inhibit some forms of fungus. Additional ingredients, such as eucalyptus, menthol, and camphor, may also have some benefits. The average time to see any improvement would be anywhere from five to sixteen months. So, patience is a virtue. Please note that the FDA does not approve Vicks VapoRub as a treatment for fungus toenails, nor does the manufacturer recommend it as a treatment.

Bleach

Adding a capful of bleach to a basin of water and soaking for about fifteen to twenty minutes a day for a couple of months may bring some change to a discolored nail. Use caution, as some people are sensitive to the bleach, and it can cause skin sensitivity or a rash.

Tea Tree Oil

A natural disinfectant, tea tree oil contains antifungal properties. Placing tea tree oil on the nail daily for at least two months may help. A complete nail cycle is one year, so be patient.

Vinegar

An antifungal remedy is just one of vinegar's 1,001 uses. Soak fungus toenails in a foot bath of equal parts vinegar and water daily for a couple of months. This is a cheap and easy way to attempt to cure a fungus nail.

Oregano Oil

Placing oregano oil on the nail two times daily for two months is a natural remedy for nail fungus. Oregano oil is extracted from the leaves of the oregano plant, and like Vicks VapoRub, contains thymol, which may be the effective ingredient. Another ingredient in oregano oil is carvacrol, which also has been shown to have antibacterial properties.

How about using antifungal topical creams?

Some topical medications are sold over-the-counter and others are by prescription. What you will find in these topical medications is an FDA-approved antifungal ingredient. Some of the more common are tolnaftate, ciclopirox, clotrimazole, econazole, miconazole, and ketoconazole. Those are some big names. There is usually one active agent in each remedy, although some topicals add additional natural antifungal ingredients such as tea tree oil.

The same elements for success apply for these topical remedies: patience, consistency, and luck. Are these medicines more effective than the home remedies? Here is the "toetal" truth: no topical agent, whether natural, home remedy, or approved nonprescription medical ingredient is very effective at eradicating toenail fungus. Toenail fungus remains difficult to treat, cure, and even improve in a good majority of cases. If you want to self-treat, choose a treatment and stick with it. If you don't see improvement, it may be time to see a podiatrist.

What will a podiatrist do at my first appointment?

At your first appointment, your podiatrist will review your medical history, ask about trauma to the foot, examine your nails, and often order a fungal culture. Nail clippings are sent to the pathology lab for evaluation. The reason for a nail culture is to determine if fungus can be isolated from the nail sample.

Even though a toenail is discolored and thick and appears to be a fungus toenail, in fact, there is a chance it may not have active fungus in the nail. This can be quite confusing for the patient. If it looks like a nail fungus and smells like a nail fungus, isn't it always a nail fungus? The answer is not always.

Some nails are damaged at the root, also called the "matrix." If the matrix has been damaged by trauma, it may be incapable of growing healthy nail. Compare this to a grey hair. Try all you might, pull it out, dye it, do whatever you can think of, and guess what? The root is only going to grow grey hair. Sometimes the nail is the same way. A damaged nail root without fungus is not uncommon. This type of nail is called a *dystrophic nail.*

If a nail culture is negative for fungus, then antifungal therapy is often ineffective. On the other hand, a positive culture confirms fungus in the toenail and also gives clues as to what may work best to cure the nail.

When the podiatrist determines I have a fungus nail, what's next?

In general, there are three treatment pathways your podiatrist may take: prescription topical antifungals, oral antifungals, and laser treatment. Let's look at each in turn.

Prescription Topicals

Depending on the case and previous care attempts, your podiatrist may recommend a prescription topical agent as a starting point for treatment. In our practice, the newest FDA-approved antifungal agents are showing significant promise over previous generations of topicals. Many patients prefer the most conservative treatment, and the topical agents are the most conservative option. Curing a toenail takes time so patients with patience get the best results. The key ingredients for success remain consistency, compliance, and luck.

Oral Medications

Next in the toolkit are the oral medications. The most common oral antifungal agent is *Lamisil,* generically called *terbinafine.* The usual prescription is one pill a day for ninety days. The oral antifungal agents have a much higher cure rate than the topical agents. If a nail culture is positive for a fungus, the medicine will clear the fungus about 60 to 70 percent of the time. Not quite a guarantee, but significantly better than topical agents.

The challenge with oral medications is the possible side effects to the liver or kidneys. Although serious side effects are rare, many patients want to avoid these oral medicines. Most podiatrists will check for a history of any liver, kidney, or medical risks including drug interactions prior to prescribing oral medications. Blood test monitoring is often used to ensure a healthy liver. Podiatrists routinely prescribe these oral medicines for their patients who are good candidates.

Laser Treatment

The laser has become a well-recognized treatment for fungus toenails. It is used to target the fungus without injuring healthy tissue surrounding the nail or beneath it. A burst of high-intensity light gently heats the toenail and alters the fungal cells, killing the toenail fungus and spores. Are you cheering? Before you plan your toenail victory party, I have to give a caveat—although the laser is a powerful tool, it can't cure all fungus toenails, yet. The results are probably similar to the oral medications, curing about two out of three patients.

The big advantage of the laser, if used correctly, is that there are no side effects. The laser requires no anesthesia and does not cause pain. There are a number of different lasers used to treat nail fungus, and technology is advancing with better and more effective lasers all the time.

Please note: Because most insurance companies do not cover laser therapy for fungus toenails, laser treatments are often an out-of-pocket cost.

Can I try several treatments at one time?

It is not uncommon for your podiatrist to "throw the book" at fungus nails and combine topical, oral, and laser treatments to eradicate fungus nails.

What about my shoes? Is the fungus living in them?

Probably. If you go through the effort to treat fungus, preventing reinfection is critical to long-term success. Fungus and bacteria can be living in the shoe and reinfect the nail. For best results when treating the toenails, also remember the shoes.

One suggestion, of course, is to get all new shoes. Another suggestion, which our office uses with great success, is a shoe sterilizer. Our favorite is ultraviolet light therapy. It kills 99.9 percent of the fungus and bacteria harbored in the shoe. This gives our patients a better chance of not getting reinfected. Simply, at the end of the day, place the ultraviolet device in your shoes and voilà! Fungus is killed. Spraying your shoes with an antifungal agent is another alternative.

So what is the future for treating fungus nails?

Although there is still no fun in fungus, there are new and more powerful lasers and more effective medications on the horizon. Although we have not won the war on fungus toenails, miracles are on the way as we advance the fight to keep your nails healthy and beautiful. Stay tuned and consult your podiatrist. Our goal is to keep you foot-loose and fungus-free!

Chapter 8
The Ingrown Nail: Cutting Corners

A toenail can turn rogue and start "growing in" on any toe at any age. I've treated tiny babies with this condition and seniors topping the century mark. Though an ingrown toenail may seem like a minor nuisance, any sufferer will tell you how painful and irritating it can be. Shoes can become near impossible to wear, and even just the pressure of the bed sheets may be difficult to bear. Far and away, the nail of the big toe is the most frequent offender, however any toenail can develop into an ingrown nail.

There are many reasons a nail may start to curve and grow into the skin alongside it, but no matter how ingrown toenails get their start, most stick around until the problem is resolved by a podiatrist. Oh, they may get better for a while, but they have the very annoying habit of returning and worsening. These chronic ingrown toenails can easily become infected.

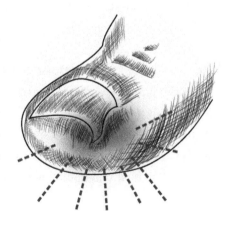

How do I know if my ingrown nail is infected?

An infected ingrown toenail becomes markedly painful, and the side of the nail is usually red and swollen, frequently with discharge. It is an acute condition, medically called a *paronychia*, and patients with infected nails should seek professional attention to eliminate pain and resolve the infection.

Parents, beware! In our office, we often see children and teenagers with festering ingrown toenails. They tend to hide their toes from their parents because they are nervous and do *not* want to go to the doctor.

Why are ingrown nails so prone to infection?

Our skin is home to all sorts of germs, and even the cleanest feet are in constant contact with bacteria. Like fungus, the bacteria thrive in the closed, warm, sweaty, dark environment of our shoes. When an ingrowing nail breaks the toe's skin, no matter how slightly, it creates a breach in the protective barrier the skin provides and opens an opportunity for the bacteria to enter and colonize the toe.

Can the infection spread?

Luckily for us, this type of infection usually stays in the toenail area and does not commonly extend past the toe. This is because the body provides a protection system around the toenail to keep the infection well localized. Of course for a diabetic, a person with poor circulation, or someone with a compromised immune system, any infection can result in serious complications and needs urgent attention.

Will I be prescribed an antibiotic?

While antibiotics may settle these infections down, they are rarely a cure. So being placed on an antibiotic, usually only helps temporarily. Removing the ingrown portion of the nail is essential to relieve infection and pain. In our office, when performing ingrown toenail removal, even for infected nails, patients often heal without the need of oral antibiotics.

Why did my nail start growing into my toe?

There are many reasons a toenail may start to turn on you. Let's take a look at some of the most common.

Heredity

Your genetic predisposition can play a big role in whether you have chronic ingrown nails. For example, a toenail may simply be too wide for the nail bed it rests on. This "wide-body" nail has nowhere to grow but into the sides of the skin. Another hereditary gift is a nail with a curved shape instead of the more usual flat shape. A curved or semicircular nail tends to put pressure on the skin edges alongside it and can develop into an ingrown nail. Over the years our nails may also change shape, starting out flat but becoming increasingly more rounded.

Thick Toenails

Unfortunately, some nails thicken over time. These thick nails may, or may not, have fungus. However, fungus is another offender that can cause ingrown nails. Thick nails tend to slowly widen. The increasing width of the nail, especially when combined with shoe pressure, can be an ingrown nail instigator.

Shoes

It doesn't take long for a tight, pointy, or narrow shoe to start to irritate toenails, or for that matter, any part of your foot. The wrong shoe can be the reason you end up at our office with a painful nail that has gone "over the edge" and needs treatment. Sometimes a new dress shoe worn to a wedding or special event is the culprit. Check out Chapter 2, "One Shoe Can Change Your Life," for some tips for picking out shoes your feet will love living in.

Athletic Shoes

Toes may feel under pressure from shoes made for a specific sports activity. For example, it is necessary for a climbing shoe to fit the foot snugly. Also a cycling shoe worn for many hours can become tight around the toes. As a foot swells in a tight shoe, the sustained pressure can cause a toenail to become ingrown and painful.

Injuries and Trauma

Here is the ugly truth about toenail trauma—it takes just one injury to damage a toenail and change how it grows forever. A nail that was once perfect can become misshapen from trauma and result in a painful ingrown nail. Just like a hair has a follicle, the nail has a root called a "matrix" that generates nail growth. A traumatic event can damage the matrix of the nail and change the nail's shape and growth pattern. Unfortunately, damage to a nail's root is not reversible. However, as we will see, ingrown toenails can be effectively treated.

Postpregnancy

Swelling in the lower extremities, increased body weight, and hormonal changes all combine to potentially affect the feet of women during and after pregnancy. A woman's foot often changes to a larger size, and ingrown toenails are not an uncommon complaint after childbirth.

Aggressive Trimming

In general, the more you trim and dig, the greater the chance of developing a painful ingrown toenail. So be gentle and go easy, less is more. If your nails are the flat type that almost never become ingrown, it is best to cut them straight across. If your nails tend to be curved on the sides but rarely get painful, you may still cut them straight across. For people who tend to get discomfort from curved or ingrowing nails, it is sometimes necessary to round the edges to give some breathing room.

Remember not to be careless when trimming, a nick with the nail clippers may become the welcome mat for a bacterial infection. For this reason, anyone who is diabetic or who has poor circulation should seek professional nail care from a local podiatrist. People with deformed nails, that may or may not be painful, certainly may find it challenging to manage their nails and may need to become a periodic visitor to the podiatrist. Foot doctors have many standing relationships with patients who need assistance with nail care.

Bathroom Surgery

Tackling your ingrown nail yourself can trap you in an endless cycle. That's what happened to my patient Ray. Every month he did battle with his ingrown toenail. He would lock the bathroom door, get out his instruments, and hack away at the nail until he felt he had pulled out the piece of toenail responsible for his pain. Often bloodied but feeling victorious, Ray would emerge from the bathroom like a warrior, proudly having conquered his ingrown nail once again. This went on until the day he lost the battle, his toe became infected, and he had to make an appointment with a podiatrist.

Many "bathroom surgeons" like Ray, reluctantly show up at our office feeling the pain of "defeet"—either their nail has become infected or the pain is too much to take. But once they realize how simple it is to permanently fix their ingrown invader, these patients ask the same question Ray did, "Why did I wait so long?" If you are waging war on an ingrown nail, it's time to call for reinforcement and let your podiatrist give you and your toe a lasting and forever peace.

What can I do at home to help my ingrown nail?

No matter what caused your ingrown toenail, there are some simple things you can do at home to help reduce pain and the risk of infection. However, if you are diabetic or have poor circulation, an immediate appointment with a podiatrist is the only recommended treatment course for you. For everyone else, here are some common at-home tips for self-care.

Soaks

Soaking your toenail in a solution of warm water and Epsom salt is an excellent way to ease discomfort. Use two teaspoons of Epsom salt in a basin of warm water. As an added benefit, Epsom salt soaks are a great way to absorb magnesium into your body. A vinegar solution is another choice for soaking a painful ingrown toenail. Use one-part white vinegar, the kind you find at the grocery store, to two-parts water. This mixture may also help to alleviate foot fungus and foot odor.

Changing Shoes

Since shoes can aggravate a toenail, changing to a different style can help. Get shoes with a wider toe box that allows more freedom for toes. Taking the pressure off nails should make it easier to navigate through the day.

Over-the-Counter Medicines

Most medications you will find on the store shelf for ingrown nails offer limited relief. The active ingredients are either topical pain relievers such as benzocaine, or gels that soften the nail in an attempt to alleviate pressure. While these medications may provide a temporary reprieve, it is imperative to understand they do not change the way the toenail grows, and your problem is likely to persist.

Topical Antibiotics

Even though these topical antiseptics may not cure an ingrown toenail, it makes sense to apply a small amount to the nail to prevent infection or limit further bacterial growth.

What about cutting a "V" in the nail or putting cotton under the nail?

There are many "old-school" remedies for ingrown toenails, and these two definitely fall into that category. When I started my practice over thirty years ago, many patients would come in saying their family doctor advised them to try one or both of these methods. I would always ask, "Did this cure your ingrown toenail?" And the answer was just about always, "No." Sometimes patients said it helped for a while, but the pain returned.

It is less common these days to see patients carve a *V* in the center of the toenail, although I do still see patients who stuff cotton under the nail. Cotton may cushion the skin and ease some discomfort; however, stuffing cotton under a corner rarely changes the way a nail grows.

When should I start to worry?

It is possible for a toenail to become ingrown just once, and with home care, tincture of time, and a little luck, you may find permanent relief. But if you have an ingrown toenail that continues to show up, causes pain in shoes, or gets red, swollen, and painful, it is time to visit your local podiatrist. A toenail that bothers you at night when the bedsheets touch it is also a sign it is time to seek professional care.

Why is a podiatrist best for treating my ingrown nail?

It's not unusual for patients with ingrown nails to be fearful and reluctant to seek help because of a painful treatment experience in their past. This is why there are specialists. One of the most rewarding and simple procedures I have provided my patients is to permanently and without any pain, relieve their ingrown toenails. Patients often say I have changed their life because the pain that had been there for so long is finally gone. If you have been avoiding treatment, don't live with the pain, seek out an experienced podiatrist. You won't be sorry!

How will my podiatrist fix my ingrown nail?

It is important to know your ingrown toenail can now be fixed with a simple pain-free, in-office procedure that takes just minutes. The other essential information is this easy procedure corrects the ingrown toenail permanently. You heard that right! It stops the nail from ingrowing ever again.

Most foot specialists perform what is called a *matrixectomy* when fixing an ingrown toenail. This technique removes the ingrown portion of the nail, and it also cauterizes the root, or matrix, to prevent that piece of ingrown nail from growing back.

This common procedure is performed in the podiatrist's office with a simple local anesthetic to numb the toe. This is one of the primary reasons to visit a podiatrist when having this procedure performed. Numbing the toe is a straightforward task that podiatrists do many times a day. With a good local anesthetic, the patient can expect a quick, easy, and totally pain-free procedure.

Your foot doctor will remove only a small amount of nail—the painful part growing under skin. Podiatrists are conscious of the long-term cosmetic result that patients want, especially women. As the area heals, the new free edge of the nail marries up nicely to the skin, so in the long term a change in appearance is barely noticeable, providing an excellent cosmetic result. Most patients can quickly return to normal activities and their shoes after an ingrown toenail correction. Home care with soaks and Band-Aid changes are done for a week or two.

And I will live happily ever after?

Well, as far as that toenail's ingrowing tendencies go, yes! Imagine the relief and joy of never having to attempt to tame that ingrown tiger in the bathroom ever again. Seek out a skilled podiatrist who can help you nail down a cure for your ingrown toenail forever. You'll be happy you did!

Chapter 9
Plantar Warts: Gone Viral?

eet get their very own kind of wart—plantar warts. These growths take up residence exclusively on the sole of the foot and vary widely in how they look and feel. Plantar warts can appear anywhere from the heel to the toe. They often begin as a raised bump that frequently gets hard and thick like a callous. Plantar warts can be single or multiple, painful or pain-free. They can grow or stay the same size, be on one foot or both feet, or spring up in clusters.

A wart is actually a virus of the *Human Papilloma Virus* (*HPV*) family. There are over one hundred different varieties of the HPV virus. A couple of them are responsible for what we commonly call plantar warts. There is much we still don't know about all types of viruses, but we do know they can be difficult to eradicate, are easily spread, and in some cases seem to stick around even after symptoms go away. Plantar warts are no exception.

How is the plantar wart virus spread?

Gyms, public pools, hotel showers, college dorms are some favorite hangouts for the virus and places where you may pick it up. Once introduced into your household, the virus can pass from one family member to another through bathroom floors and showers.

Parents, beware! There are no reliable studies addressing the frequency of plantar warts or whose feet they favor most, but it is estimated that 10 to 20 percent of all children and adolescents at some point find this unwelcome visitor camped out on the bottom of their foot.

If I come into contact with the virus, will I definitely get warts?

No. It *is* possible to come into contact with a plantar wart and not get the virus. We are all individuals with unique immune systems. Some people who come into contact with a common cold virus succumb, and others don't. It's the same with warts. You may have an immune system that is stronger or one that is more resistant to the plantar wart virus.

If I avoid public showers and other places the virus is likely to lurk, can I prevent getting plantar warts?

If you avoid these places, you will be less likely to get the virus, but keeping your feet away from shared bathrooms is no guarantee. Viruses are still a bit mysterious to us, but one theory holds that they remain inside of our bodies and can show up unexpectedly, without any warning. In fact, it is not uncommon for me to see a patient who lives a private lifestyle, has excellent hygiene, is never at a gym or public pool, does not live with anyone with warts, and has, all of sudden, a wart pop up on a foot. You may be harboring a dormant plantar wart virus that decides to become active and express itself on your foot at any time.

I stepped on something, hurt my foot, and now I have a wart there.

I have heard many a patient relate a story of stepping on an object and then feeling something on the bottom of their foot months later in the exact same spot. Often the patient thinks a bit of the object is embedded in the foot, only to discover it is a plantar wart. Why does this happen? The skin acts as a barrier to outside intruders. An abrasion or tiny opening is all the opportunistic wart virus may need to invade and set up shop on your foot.

I started with one wart, now I have a lot of them.

It is not unusual to start with one wart and end up with multiple warts on the bottom of both feet. Young people most commonly experience multiplying warts; however, it can be quite disheartening for anyone to have a colony of warts show up where there should be no trespassing allowed.

The Mother Wart

If there are multiple warts, the first to appear is often called "the mother." As the virus spreads, additional warts are described as satellites or baby warts. Most foot specialists recommend treating a wart at first sight to prevent it spreading to new places on your feet and to prevent passing it on to others. Parents take note!

Mosaic Warts

A variation of the common plantar wart, mosaic warts grow in clusters on the bottom of the foot and tend to take up a large surface area. These warts are very active and seem to spread and enlarge faster than common plantar warts.

Will my wart spread if I don't treat it?

Not all warts multiply. Sometimes a patient ventures into the office to have a growth evaluated that has been on a foot for quite some time. Often they are surprised to find out that the lesion is indeed a plantar wart that has never grown larger, become painful, or spread to other areas.

Can a plantar wart be cancerous?

It is rare to have a cancer or melanoma in the foot—however, it is important for any growth to be evaluated. The average person cannot differentiate between a wart and a suspicious lesion, so a dangerous growth can go untreated and undiagnosed.

One of my patients, Sarah, came into the office with a lesion on the bottom of her foot that she thought was a plantar wart. Sarah had discovered the "wart" some time ago, but noticed that it had become larger. The growth turned out not to be a wart. Unfortunately, it was a cancerous melanoma. Thankfully, with aggressive treatment, this wonderful person is still around to talk about it.

Please don't take the chance of mistaking a serious condition for a wart. It is safest to have a podiatrist evaluate any growth on your foot. And if you get a diagnosis of warts, keep a watchful eye on them. If they change in size or color or discomfort, it's best to seek additional treatment.

When should I see a podiatrist about my plantar wart?

I recommend seeing a podiatrist to get a diagnosis when you first discover any growth. As we discussed above, other conditions can be mistaken for warts and warts for other conditions. This is the challenge with warts. They do need a proper diagnosis. See a podiatrist to determine whether you have a plantar wart—even if you are thinking of self-treating the wart at home.

How will a podiatrist diagnose the wart?

Warts in general have a characteristic appearance that podiatrists are quick to recognize. The wart usually has little black dots in its center that are tiny capillaries indicative of the wart virus. Warts have their own unique blood supply, which is probably how they travel around and spread so well. Upon trimming a wart down, the podiatrist looks for what we call pinpoint capillary hemorrhaging. These small dots of blood help in diagnosis of the plantar wart.

If the podiatrist thinks any growth is suspicious, he or she will remove and biopsy it to ensure it is, in fact, benign.

Can plantar warts go away on their own?

A percentage of warts, if given enough time, resolve on their own. However, many warts, if left alone, stay, spread, and get bigger.

So, how do you know what to do? It depends on a few factors. Is the wart painful? Is it getting bigger? Is it sticking around and not shrinking in size? Are you concerned about it being contagious and spreading to other family members? If you answer yes to any of the above, or just want to get rid of it, see a podiatrist.

Are there home treatments I can try?

There are many home-remedy success stories about plantar warts. However, they are anecdotal. This does not mean home remedies don't work. It just means there is no medical basis or supported study for any particular home treatment. The success rate of any home treatment yields probably the same results as giving a plantar wart time to go away on its own.

If you decide you want to give a home remedy a try, I describe some of the most popular below.

Over-the-Counter Wart Medicines

These OTC medications are usually a mild salicylic acid preparation used to soften and remove layers of skin in an attempt to resolve the wart. They can either be a liquid you put on directly or embedded in a patch that is placed on the wart. Both forms usually require a daily application and also a periodic scraping to get the previously applied medicine off and the new medicine directly on the wart. For children, the medicine can be put on at bedtime, making it easy for a parent to apply. Home treatment should be limited to a few weeks unless you are under a doctor's supervision to evaluate for progress.

Freezing the Wart

Another over-the-counter option is freezing the wart. Freeze kits are available for home treatment, and although they do not contain liquid nitrogen, which is what the specialist uses, these freeze techniques can sometimes be successful.

Duct Tape

If you want to give this a go, keep the wart covered with duct tape day in and day out for about six days. Then remove the tape, soak the wart, use an emery board or scrape the wart down, and repeat. Do this consistently for about a month. Why does it work? No one knows for sure, but it may trigger an immune response that helps the body fight the wart virus. Keeping the wart dry and covered may help too. Either way, this is a pretty safe home remedy to try.

Natural Treatments

Many home remedies for plantar warts have been passed down through generations and are made of an array of ingredients that are applied directly to the wart. Although there are minimal side effects, any of these can cause localized irritation or burning on the skin. To be clear, I am not recommending a specific treatment. If after a few weeks there is no response, it is time to seek other remedies. Here are a few natural ingredients to consider:

- Crushed vitamin C in a paste
- Crushed garlic
- Potato (yes a potato slice) applied to the wart
- Zinc ointment
- Dandelion

Who should not self-treat?

Any person who has diabetes, poor circulation, a history of skin cancer, or difficulty healing cuts or wounds should only seek professional care and avoid self-treatment. Also self-treatment should be attempted only if you are confident the lesion is in fact a plantar wart.

When is it time to give up on a home remedy?

If your wart is going to respond to home treatment, it should do so within a month. If it doesn't, then you probably have a stubborn and resistant wart that likes its home and thinks it has squatter's rights. In this case, it is time to visit your local foot specialist and have it treated professionally.

How will a podiatrist treat my wart?

After confirming a diagnosis of a plantar wart, your podiatrist has a range of treatments to offer. What treatment plan is best for you will depend on your situation. Your age, activity level, and occupation factor in, as well as specifics about your wart—how large it is, where it is located on the foot, whether it is in a prime weight-bearing spot, and how many warts you have. Taking all this into consideration, your podiatrist can help you weigh the pros and cons of each option and make a recommendation. This could be a brand-new laser, a new freezing technique, or a magic medicine that makes warts say "Uncle!" with just two or three treatments. I describe some of the most widely used treatments for plantar warts below.

Chemical Cauterization

Every podiatrist has his or her favorite medical-grade medication to apply to plantar warts. The medicine the doctor uses is much stronger than what is commercially available over-the-counter. After initial application of the medicine, the typical regimen is a visit every two weeks to remove more of the wart that is dying off and to apply new medicine to destroy any remaining wart. Although this method may require a number of office visits to resolve your wart, this treatment is usually painless, which also makes it a good option for children. If a doctor uses the stronger medicines, a blister may form, and the wart may fall off with the blister.

Laser Treatments

Special lasers can be used to treat and remove warts. An example is the Nd:YAG laser, which has the added benefit of requiring no anesthesia for treatment. This particular laser effectively targets the blood supply of warts to eradicate them. Laser wart treatment is performed only if the specialist has a laser in-office.

Cryotherapy

In this treatment, the wart is frozen with liquid nitrogen. New cryosurgery units offer improved treatment success over some of the previous generation of freezing techniques. The liquid nitrogen freezes the skin and then a blister forms, and the wart falls off with the blister. Multiple treatments may be necessary for stubborn warts. The thickness of the skin on the bottom of the foot can limit the success of cryotherapy.

Surgery

There are benefits and drawbacks to surgically removing warts. On the plus side, the warts are out and gone in one visit. On the downside, the site may take up to a couple of weeks to heal, and depending on the size and location of the wart, can be quite annoying as it mends.

Parents, beware! Because the area needs to be anesthetized this may not be the best choice for a child.

Injections of Medicine

In difficult-to-eradicate cases, a treatment option may be to inject the wart with a strong medicine such as *bleomycin* to resolve the wart. This medicine is also used for chemotherapy and can be highly effective for the most resistant and challenging warts.

Drying Agents

Many podiatrists attack moisture on sweaty feet to create a less friendly environment for warts. Medicines that essentially act as antiperspirants for the feet are prescribed for daily use in tandem with other common wart treatments.

Is my wart gone for good?

Successful treatment of a plantar wart does not guarantee you will never get another wart. Remember, the wart is a virus. It may go away forever, or it may be scared off into hiding until further notice.

For best long-term results, keep your immune system strong, practice good hygiene, avoid being barefoot in public places, and inspect your feet regularly. Have family members with warts use their own towels and spray the tub with a disinfectant. If a wart shows up, don't let it get under your skin, see a podiatrist.

Chapter 10

Bunions: Beyond the Bump

B unions can sneak up on you quietly over time. One day you look down, and lo and behold, where your own foot used to be, you now see your grandma's. There is a bump just like hers sticking out on the side of the foot, near the big toe. And that big toe doesn't look so straight anymore. It is angling over toward the second toe.

The "bump" is the bunion, and as time goes by it may protrude more and more from the side of the foot. It can become quite painful and make finding a comfortable shoe difficult. Interestingly, size does not always matter when it comes to bunion pain. A small bunion may be extremely painful, and a large one not bother the foot owner at all.

Sadly, past generations suffered with their bunions or underwent surgeries that had poor cosmetic outcomes and often did not prevent the bunion from recurring. But today we have techniques that can give bunion patients excellent results—a fully functioning, pain-free, bump-free, and permanently corrected foot!

Why do I have a bunion?

People have a predisposition for bunions based on heredity. If Mom or Dad or Grandma had bunions, you may get to have them too. Most bunion sufferers have inherited a foot type that slowly develops an instability surrounding the great toe joint. Foot specialists have studied the foot's complex biomechanics, including muscle, tendon, ligament, and bone function, to understand how and why a bunion advances. Thankfully, in today's world if you suffer from bunion pain and deformity, you have first-rate options for relief.

Parents, beware! Bunions are not solely for the mature. Although bunions most commonly show up in our thirties or forties, sometimes the hereditary influence can start in the early teen years. Some teens rapidly develop bunions and require treatment.

Did my shoes cause my bunion?

Believe it or not, wearing the "wrong" shoes is not a primary reason for developing bunions. Shoes with a narrow or pointy toe box can make a bunion hurt a whole lot more and can speed the formation of a bunion, but shoes are not the cause of bunions in the great majority of cases.

How do we know shoes alone do not cause bunions? Studies of African tribal groups who have never worn shoes revealed that these groups have bunions at the same rate as shoe wearers, even though they may never have donned a shoe or a high heel! Please understand, this is not a license from the foot doctor to wear pointy, narrow shoes. I share the study results just to help you understand that even if you own only smart and sensible shoes, you can still develop a bunion if it is in your family tree.

Will my bunion grow?

Bunion

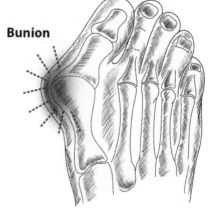

Most of my patients think the bone in their foot becomes larger and grows a "bunion" on it. This is not the case. The bunion "bump" is not truly a growth of bone. What actually happens as a bunion develops is the first metatarsal bone (there are five), which spans the arch and connects to the big toe, starts to angle away from the foot. As the metatarsal bone pivots farther out, the bunion increases in size, usually slowly over time. This action then causes a reaction: the big toe moves in the opposite direction, toward the other toes. Slowly, the bunion gets bigger on the side of the foot, and slowly the big toe encroaches on the second toe.

Is the bump on the other side of my foot a bunion?

A bump that protrudes on the outside of the foot just behind the "pinky" toe is called a tailor's bunion, also known as a mini bunion or a bunionette. The bump belongs to the fifth metatarsal bone, and like the more common big toe bunion, in most cases it is not an extra growth of bone but the result of a change in the position of the bone. Slowly over time, the fifth metatarsal bone spreads or splays outward, away from the foot, and a bump begins to appear. The pinky toe may also move inward toward the other toes.

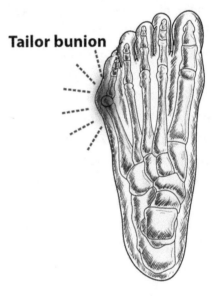

Tailor bunion

The tailor's bunion got its name from old-time tailors who used the outside of their foot to continually press the sewing pedal. The repetitive stress and microtrauma often irritated the bone, and so, the name tailor's bunion came to be. Most tailor's bunions nowadays are not caused by trauma; they are caused by a hereditary predisposition.

A protruding tailor's bunion can often be painful, or it can live peacefully without causing discomfort. Much depends on shoe choice, occupation, activity level, size of the tailor's bunion, and if the nerve or soft tissue surrounding the area becomes irritated. Treatment options are the same as for the "big toe" bunion, so read on!

Is there anything I can do at home to treat my bunion?

Unfortunately, options for improving bunions are limited. You either live with a bunion or have it fixed surgically. Certainly, there are a number of ways to help bunions be more comfortable. Most of these conservative remedies are designed to take the pressure off the bunion bump so it doesn't rub and get irritated in the shoe.

Shoe Strategies

Ditch the pinchers. First and foremost, get rid of shoes that cause pain and irritate your bunion. If you do not have the heart to throw away your painful shoes, place them in a box marked "Do Not Wear" in the back of your closet. Better yet, donate them to a worthy charity or sell them on eBay to someone who doesn't have a bunion

Go boxy. Change your shoe style to shoes with a wider toe box. Think Volvo—boxy is good and safe. Make sure the shoe material directly over the bunion is soft and does not have any seams to irritate the bunion. Soft, wide, and roomy are the keys to comfort for bunion sufferers. For those who are lucky enough to live in warm weather year-round, open-toed shoes and sandals are a wonderful way to keep your bunion happy. Of course, your bunion is now exposed for the world to see, but it beats throbbing inside your shoe.

Switch it up. Changing shoes frequently is another strategy. Each shoe fits differently, so changing shoes is a relief for feet. I often recommend having two pairs of shoes with you. When one pair becomes painful, switch to the other.

Cushioning

Pads and bunion protectors may offer some relief. Made out of materials like gel, silicone, or foam, the pads are used mostly to cushion the bunion and relieve pressure.

Topicals

Temporary pain relief is just the ticket for that occasionally painful bunion. Although everyone has their favorite topical (or whatever may be in the medicine chest or drawer), here are a few options:

- *Topricin*: One of my favorite topicals. Contains many natural and effective anti-inflammatories and pain relievers. Good for sore muscles and joints too.
- *Arnica*: This is a fan favorite of many, especially in holistic communities.
- *Biofreeze*: A blast of cold and a temporary deep freeze help soothe the pain.
- *Lidocaine creams or patches*: Sometimes a little numbing agent helps.
- *Capsaicin creams*: The ingredient found in hot peppers can afford relief by stimulating, then decreasing the pain intensity.
- *Voltaren gel*: A topical nonsteroidal anti-inflammatory. Requires a prescription.

Splints and Braces

Don't expect a splint or a brace to correct a bunion deformity. They may help limit progression and ease some discomfort. For maximum benefit, it's best to start at the first sign of a bunion. The bigger the bunion, the less responsive it is and the less likely the splint or brace will help slow bunion growth.

Is there anything a podiatrist can do without surgery to relieve my bunion?

A painful bunion may be helped by a steroid injection. Sometimes a nerve that courses over the bunion becomes inflamed and irritated. Depositing a local anesthetic with a corticosteroid may relieve pain.

Also, there can be inflammation directly over the bunion resulting in soft tissue swelling. This is often called a bursal sac or bursitis over the bunion bump. An injection may help reduce soft tissue swelling and pain.

In addition to the painful bunion bump, the joint itself can become inflamed and develop intra-articular pain, or arthritis of varying degree. (We'll talk about this more later in the chapter and also in Chapter 17 on arthritis.) A cortisone injection can reduce pain that stems from arthritis inside the joint.

Although injections are not a cure for your bunion, they can provide relief for a short or even extended period of time. Some podiatrists may attempt an injection to help put off surgery for their patients, while others go directly to surgery without passing go. There is no right or wrong answer, as it depends on the patient, the bunion, and the pain.

Custom Orthotics:

Podiatrists often fit a patient with custom orthotics to help slow down bunion development. Orthotics can alter improper foot function such as excessive pronation, potentially slowing the bunion progression while providing comfort to the foot. This is a favorite treatment for young patients showing early signs of bunion growth and for those who are not yet ready for surgery.

Is surgery the best option?

Surgery is the only way to correct a bunion deformity, but that does not mean it is the best option for you. Consult with a foot surgeon to discuss your particular case. At the first appointment, the surgeon will perform an evaluation, take x-rays, and discuss your pain level and previous attempts at conservative treatment. The x-rays and exam are the important factors for deciding if you are a good candidate for surgery, but, of course, there are many additional factors your surgeon will consider, including your age, medical history, occupation, goals, and more.

How do I pick a surgeon?

How to choose a foot surgeon is discussed in detail in Chapter 20. All surgeons are not created equal, and selecting a skilled foot surgeon is crucial for success. Here let me remind you that board certification, routine performance of the procedure you are having done, recommendations from staff, positive word of mouth in your community, and happy patients are all good indicators of a skilled surgeon.

What will my x-rays tell the surgeon?

In reviewing x-rays, surgeons focus on the critical factor we call the *intermetatarsal angle*. This angle is a measure of how far the first metatarsal bone has moved away from the second metatarsal bone.

The greater the angle, the more advanced the bunion deformity. A normal angle would measure between 5 and 10 degrees. A mild to moderate bunion may measure up to 14 degrees, and a severe bunion may measure greater than 14 degrees. Severity can determine what type of surgery is needed and thus, recovery time postprocedure.

So I should have surgery sooner than later?

Without question, it is easier for our patients to have their bunions corrected before they get to the severe stages. But we do not always operate in the early stages. The bunion may not be painful, the patient may not be a good candidate for surgery because of other health issues, or the timing may not be right for the patient. Surgery always has risks, and we only operate when the benefit to the patient outweighs them.

My grandma said her bunion came back after surgery.

Thankfully, the advances in bunion surgery have been fantastic. Modern, leading-edge procedures not only provide pain relief and a good cosmetic result, they also hold up for the long term and consider the important functional requirements for today's active lifestyles.

Fifty years ago, we did not understand the importance of the mechanics of the foot and how it functioned internally. Surgeons "correcting" bunions did not address the intermetatarsal angle. They simply shaved off the bunion "bump" and called it a day. This only removed the bunion temporarily. In many cases, the bunion returned because the underlying problem of the metatarsal bone moving away was not corrected.

"Back in the day," surgeons would also sometimes remove the big toe joint, which often left the patient with a short toe and a nonfunctional joint. Surgical techniques were more primitive decades ago. Today, performing this procedure would be potential grounds for malpractice, yet back then it was done routinely. But those days are gone! With the terrific advances both in understanding bunions and the surgical procedures to correct them, you can expect a functioning foot without recurrence of your bunion. It is now possible to escape your inheritance of painful feet!

Bunions: A Family Affair

When Taylor came to the office with her mom at age seventeen complaining of a painful bunion, she was the third generation in her family to seek correction at our practice. Her grandma was first, about twenty-five years prior, followed by her mom, and now Taylor. Each of them had a different stage of bunion development when they came in for treatment. Grandma had the severe "grandma" bunion, mom had a moderate deformity, and Taylor's was now suddenly growing larger and hurting when she played sports and wore most shoes. As they say, the apple doesn't fall far from the tree. Heredity played a large role in this family's foot problems, but thankfully, all now successfully sport feet without bunions. Of course, they were all given the podiatrist spiel about practical shoes and being smart with shoe choices, but mostly they wear any shoes they want and have no pain.

How will the foot surgeon fix my bunion?

There are many procedures and techniques for correcting bunions. Your foot surgeon will decide which state-of-the-art procedure is best for you. Evaluation will include

- size and stage of your bunion,
- if there is painful joint involvement,
- range of motion of the joint,
- whether the deformity is stiff and rigid or loose and hypermobile,
- whether you have additional deformities, such as hammer toes or calluses on the ball of your foot, and
- pain level.

As surgeons, we also want to get to know you before making a procedure recommendation. What kind of shoes do you expect to wear long-term? Are you a marathon runner or more of a couch potato? We want to know if you will be compliant in the postsurgical period and follow directions to ensure healing, and what your expectations are. Do you understand you cannot resume Zumba classes the week after; that if the bunion is on your right foot, you will not be able to drive for a period of time; and that if you have little kids, you may need some help around the house?

The Austin Bunionectomy for Mild to Moderate Bunions

The *Austin bunionectomy* was not named after Austin, Texas. It was named after a foot surgeon named Dale Austin, who first published his findings in 1981. Since then, the Austin bunionectomy has become the procedure of choice for many foot surgeons for the correction of mild to moderate bunions. In fact, some surgeons choose this procedure even for severe bunions, if the patient cannot be on crutches and requires a speedier return to weight bearing, usually within a week or two.

Typically, one or two screws are used to hold the correction. Screws usually remain in the foot after surgery. They rarely, if ever, bother a patient and basically become part of the bone. One cannot usually feel them, and because the materials are inert, they rarely cause any reactions. You can still get through TSA without the alarms going off, so no worry there either.

Procedures for Severe Bunions

Severe bunions with high intermetatarsal angles may require a different procedure from an Austin bunionectomy. Depending on the surgeon's preference either a *Lapidus bunionectomy* or a *base wedge osteotomy* are commonly performed to correct the severe bunion. The same modern fixation techniques are used as in the Austin bunionectomy; however, because procedures for severe bunions are done near the base of the metatarsal bone, early weight bearing can create complications and jeopardize the desired result. Patients often must limit weight bearing for four to eight weeks to allow for full stability of the surgical area during healing.

A Bunion plus Arthritis

The garden-variety bunions that we see day-to-day in the office usually are not arthritic. However, arthritis in the big toe joint, medically known as *hallux limitus* or *hallux rigidus*, is another common cause of pain around this area. Someone with a bona fide bunion may also at times have arthritis in the joint—a double treat! Arthritis develops as a result of a wearing away of the joint surfaces between two bones and is commonly caused by either a hereditary predisposition or trauma.

If there is arthritis in or around your joint and this is the primary cause of your pain, there are specific procedures to eliminate joint pain. These may include removing bone spurs and joint cleanup for the early arthritic joints, and either fusions or joint implants for the more advanced arthritic deformities. See Chapter 17 for more about arthritis and its treatment.

Osteotomy for Tailor's Bunions

An *osteotomy* is a precisely placed surgical cut into the bone to allow for realignment and repositioning of the fifth metatarsal bone. By performing an osteotomy in an exact manner, we can ensure the bone is positioned and relocated in an optimal place to relieve pain and also prevent a return of the tailor's bunion. This provides a long-lasting correction and a good cosmetic result.

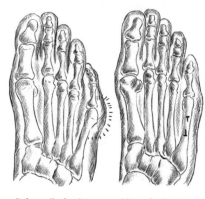

Before tailor bunion
correction

After tailor bunion
correction

Not Your Grandma's Bunion

Bunions are game changers (and shoe changers) for those who suffer with pain. Today's advances in surgical techniques have allowed bunions to be corrected with more precision and provide excellent results both functionally and cosmetically. So, now there is no reason to grow up like Grandma anymore. Visit your foot surgeon for a consultation, and see if saying bye-bye to bunion blues is right for you.

Chapter 11

Hammer Toes:
Bent out of Shape

I n a perfect world, everyone has ten beautifully straight toes. In the real world, a whole lot of people don't. Toes that become bent at the knuckle and are no longer straight are called hammer toes. Approximately 60 million people suffer from hammer toes in the United States alone.

The middle three toes are the most susceptible to becoming permanently bent, and the problem is not just a cosmetic one. Hammer toes interfere with foot function. They are also painful. Fortunately, we have tried-and-true surgical procedures to correct crooked toes, and almost 550,000 surgeries are performed annually to bring relief to those who suffer from this condition.

Why did I get a hammer toe?

Heredity often plays a large role in many of the medical conditions we develop, and you can add hammer toes to the list. Though we are not born with hammer toes, the mechanics of our own particular feet may lead to them developing over time. Specifically, the action of the toe tendons and attached muscles has the most influence on whether or not we get hammer toes.

Tendons course along both the top and bottom of the toes. The top tendons are called the *extensor tendons*, and the tendons on the bottom of the toes are called the *flexor tendons*. In perfect toes, the flexor and extensor tendons perform their jobs dutifully to bend our toes upward or downward. As we walk, the tendons help create a balance where the toes are stabilized on the ground and provide a lever to walk forward.

However, in certain feet, one of the tendons may exert more of a force than the other. If, for example, the bottom tendon applies more downward pull, this naturally starts the process of a toe becoming slightly bent. As we experience this "overpulling" of the tendon for thousands of steps every day, every week, every month, year after year, the toe eventually takes on the bent shape permanently and, voilà, it is an official full-time hammer toe.

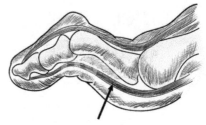

Hammer toe due to overpulling of the flexor tendon

Does wearing the wrong shoes play a role?

Yes. While shoes are rarely the sole cause of a hammer toe, the wrong shoes often play a role in hastening the development of a bent toe.

What happens? Well, shoes that are too small, narrow, or pointy cram your toes so they are not free to move about. Think airline seats and being wedged into the middle seat with no elbow or leg room for hours on end, day after day. Not fun, not comfy. Now imagine tilting that middle airline seat forward so you are bent over. That's how toes feel when high heels push them into a "downward dog" yoga position and keep them there all day. Forcing your feet into an anatomically incorrect position speeds up the development of the deformity.

My advice: when in the shoe store, admire but leave the pretty, painful shoe for someone else. As the saying goes, "Buyer, beware," or in this case "Buyer, don't wear!"

Are there other causes of hammer toes?

A broken toe or a bunion deformity can cause a hammer toe. Let's look at how each of these events may end up leading a straight toe astray.

Bunions

When a bunion forms, the big toe moves in toward the second toe, pushing the second toe aside and often causing it to become hammered. Poor Number 2! This can start a domino effect as each toe pushes the next, turning even third and fourth toes into hammer toes. For more about how bunions form and treatments to correct them, see Chapter 10.

Broken toes

A toe injury, especially a broken toe, is often the cause of a solitary hammer toe. When it comes to a broken toe, people often think, "There is nothing to do about it so why get it looked at?" Well, here's the answer straight from the Foot Doctor: you get it looked at so you don't develop a painful hammer toe, an arthritic toe, or a bone spur. For toe fractures, the podiatrist will make sure the toe has the best chance of healing in the correct position with the least chance of a developing a problem down the road. Broken toe treatment is discussed in more detail in Chapter 16.

My toe is bent, but I can push on the joint and straighten it. Is it a hammer toe?

Probably. Hammer toes come in different varieties. The middle toes—toes two, three, and four—each has three bones (phalanges) that are connected by two joints. The classic hammer toe is a buckling or bending of the first joint, the one closer to the foot. It can be either flexible or rigid.

If you have a *flexible hammer toe*, as the name indicates, the toe can be straightened but bounces back. Usually, flexible hammer toes are not terribly painful, because when the shoe hits the top of the toe, the toe is able to move out of the way.

A *rigid hammer toe*, on the other hand, cannot be straightened when you push on it. It is fixed in the deformed and bent position. Most hammer toes begin as the flexible type and with time change into the more severe rigid variety. We see lots of flexible and rigid hammer toes in our office, but we fix rigid toes more frequently because they are more painful and patients need relief.

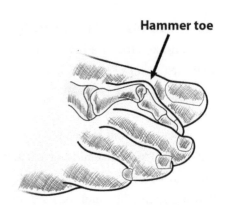

Hammer toe

What about mallet toes? What are they?

There are two other types of bent toes, the *mallet toe* and the *claw toe*. If the second joint of the toe, the one nearest the toe's end, bends or buckles that is classically called a "mallet toe." If both the toe joints are bent or buckled, that is typically referred to as a "claw toe." So we have a hammer, a mallet, and a claw. Not words you ever want associated with your toes!

In most cases, the hammer toe takes top billing, as it is the most common deformity. It also has become the de facto terminology used by physicians and patients alike regardless of whether a mallet or a claw is a more correct anatomical name for the toe in question.

Why do I have a painful corn on my hammer toe?

If you have a hammer toe, you may soon find you also have a painful corn. As the toe joint buckles up and the shoe presses on the knuckle, the skin on the knuckle begins to thicken in response to the increased friction and pressure. Just like you get calluses on your hands from raking leaves all day, your toe gets a corn from rubbing against your shoe. Some of these corns develop a deep-seated core that often inflames and irritates the skin surrounding the corn and becomes extremely painful.

If I get rid of the corn, will I get rid of my problem?

Many people believe if you remove the corn you have fixed the toe. This is not the case. Removing the corn affords temporary pain relief. However, the corn in most cases will return because the hammer toe is still present. So treating the corn is a big help for pain relief, but not a cure, especially if you do not modify your shoes.

Why is the tip of my toe painful?

A hammer toe may also put extra pressure on the tip of the toe. The body reacts to the repeated pressure by forming a corn. These hard corns at the toe's tip can be quite painful and require treatment.

I'm getting corns between my toes.

Corns between toes are not uncommon with hammer toes. When anything is stressed it grows. When muscles are stressed they get bigger. When the stomach is stressed, it gets bigger. Well, when the bone in the joint of the hammer toe is stressed by chronic friction, it may get bigger too. The bone's response to the pressure is to grow a bone spur. These bony outcroppings can rub against a neighboring toe, and the friction can cause a painful corn to form. These inter-toe corns are called "soft" corns, although they may not feel at all soft!

What's up with my pinky toe? It's curly and has corns.

The fifth toe frequently does not sit straight. It can range from being just a bit curly to being so rotated it sits on its side and you cannot even see the toenail as you look down. Pinky toes, whether curly, rotated, or bent, all fall under the category of hammer toes. Maybe the curly toe was helpful in climbing trees when we were forest dwellers, but because we now wear shoes, pinky toes often get rubbed the wrong way.

It is not uncommon for me to see patients who complain that even the littlest corn on the fifth toe is one of the most painful conditions they can remember experiencing. These painful corns can be found inside the toe where it rubs on the fourth toe, or outside the toe where it rubs on the shoe. Often a bone spur forms in response to chronic irritation and pressure and is the underlying cause of the toe pain. The little toe can make some big noise when it is angry with you for choosing the wrong footwear!

Evolutionists say that in future generations the little toe may be a thing of the past, but for now those painful pinky toes may have your attention.

The ball of my foot hurts and I have hammer toes—are the two related?

Very likely. Remember the law of physics that states for every action there is an equal and opposite reaction? Well, in this case, as the hammer toe begins to buckle upward, the adjoining metatarsal bone is forced downward. The normal toe position is end to end where the base of the toe meets the adjoining metatarsal.

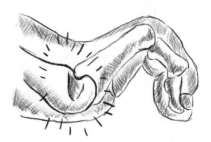

However, as the deformity develops, the toe bone starts to sit more on top of the metatarsal bone, and this joint may begin to subtly dislocate downward. As it advances, the condition is called *predislocation syndrome*, or *PDS*, and the metatarsal starts to "drop," putting more pressure on the ball of the foot. At

Hammer toe causing painful metatarsal

this point, you may develop pain or callouses or both. So a hammer toe can most definitely cause pain in the ball of the foot.

What can I do to home-treat my hammer toe?

The first treatment to try for painful hammer toes is to change your shoe style. You may have already done this without success, but did you get a wider shoe? A shoe with a higher toe box? A completely different style? A full or half size larger?

If you have tried moving your toes into bigger or better shoes and they still hurt, there are other home remedies. Most of these are designed to separate the toes, reduce the friction from the shoe, or reduce the painful corn. Attempting these treatments may give relief; however, without a long-term shoe modification, the relief may be short-lived.

Buyer, beware! Home treatment for corns and hammer toes is a huge business, with drug stores and supermarkets devoting significant shelf space to products. As you will learn below, some medicated products are *not safe*, particularly for people who have diabetes or poor circulation, and some tools pose infection risks.

Separation

For "soft" corns between toes, separating the toes reduces the friction and relieves pain. You can start with simple Vaseline. Apply a generous amount between the painful toes. If that doesn't do the trick, cotton or lamb's wool is a good choice to reduce friction and keep toes apart. There are also small pads designed to sit between toes and stop them from rubbing. Usually made of a soft foam, felt, or gel, they are a simple way to get some relief.

Cushioning

For "hard" corns or pain on the top of the toe, pads are used to off-load the painful area. They are usually designed with a hole that is placed over the corn. A Band-Aid over the pad holds it in place for the day. Gel pads slipped onto the toe are popular and effective pain relievers. The gel absorbs the shoe shock. For corns on the tip of the toe, there are "buttress," or "crest," pads that are designed to fit under the toes to relieve the pressure points. Finding the pad that works best is often a matter of trial and error. But it's best to experiment with these simple pads and avoid the medicated kind discussed below.

Corn Removers

These medicated over-the-counter products contain an ingredient, often a salicylic acid preparation, that eats away at the corn. It can come in a liquid or be embedded in a pad. These products always have a warning, but in very tiny print that you may not notice. Here is my warning: If you are a diabetic or have poor circulation, do not use corn-removing products. The acid they contain will not distinguish between a corn and normal skin. We foot specialists see emergencies on a regular basis because the medicated pads burn through the skin and create a nasty wound or infection. In general, most foot specialists do not recommend these products because of the complications we see when not used properly, but they remain readily available on store shelves.

Filing versus Cutting

Softening and filing corns down is the safest way to remove corns on your own. Soften the corn first by soaking the foot for fifteen to twenty minutes. Then remove the hard skin over the corn with a file or emery board. You can also use your fingers to peel off any skin that you can remove safely.

There are skin peelers commercially available to peel or pare down calluses and corns. Sometimes they look like a cheese grater and some have a sharp blade. Using a blade on your corns can be technically difficult and, just like shaving, can result in nicks, cuts, and bleeding. Because corns are tucked in awkward places like between your toes, they are hard to see and get at. "Oops!" is a common exclamation for bathroom surgeons. And because even clean feet have a multitude of bacteria and fungi living on them, infection is a risk. Every podiatrist can share disaster stories, including loss of a toe or toes, from infection. **Diabetics or anyone with less than perfect circulation, sensation, or eyesight should only see a foot specialist for foot care**.

If you choose to self-treat in this fashion, please use caution, and seek a foot specialist's help if the pain does not subside.

Prevention

Wearing comfortable shoes with plenty of toe room is the best prevention. Remember that shoes that push and bend toes advance the deformity faster. I also recommend calf stretching. If the calf muscles are tight (often called *equinus deformity*), this can cause the small muscles and tendons of the foot to compensate, and toe deformities can advance over time. So calf stretching can be helpful. For early onset flexible hammer toes, stretching your toes upward may be helpful to relax tight tendons and slow development.

Orthotics may be helpful as well. These specialty inserts designed from a cast of your foot are placed in your shoe to improve foot function by reducing strain and keeping the toe tendons from overpulling. Good shoes, stretching, and orthotics are the best bets to prevent or slow hammer toe development.

When is it time to seek professional help from a podiatrist?

Most people recognize a hammer toe and feel the effects of a painful corn. If shoe changes and home treatments have not relieved your pain, it's time to visit a podiatrist. A first appointment with a foot specialist begins with an examination and x-rays. Then your foot doctor can review your options. These fall into two categories: conservative treatment and surgical correction.

What are the options for conservative treatment?

Removal of your painful corns and a plan to protect your toes from continued aggravation are the components of conservative treatment. Many patients who choose conservative care are seen regularly in the office to relieve painful corns. This is an acceptable and common way to maintain comfort that can last anywhere from a month to a year or more. It all depends on the severity of your toe deformity, your activity level, and type of shoes you wear. Eventually, a pattern is observed, and patients either schedule regular appointments for corn removal or call when pain relief is needed.

So how will the doctor remove my corns?

Carefully, of course. Podiatrists use specialty instruments and usually soften corns for a few minutes before paring them down. This can be accomplished in most cases without any discomfort. If necessary, depending on the location and pain associated with the corn, the toe can be anesthetized to make it easier to allow for pain-free corn removal.

Sometimes a small amount of an anti-inflammatory is injected along with the anesthetic to reduce soft tissue inflammation caused by the hammer toe. Relief is immediate and happy patients are returned to pain-free living.

It is important to recognize corn removal by the podiatrist is not a cure for your hammer toe, and the pain can readily return. Many people think that just getting a corn removed cures the toe; however, the underlying hammer toe deformity is not corrected simply by relieving a painful corn.

The foot doctor usually makes shoe recommendations and offers pads for use between visits. Many podiatrists have an in-office dispensary of the best and most commonly used pads to help keep your toes pain-free for as long as possible.

When should I consider surgery?

Toes are often so bent out of shape or so painful that conservative care does not provide long-term pain relief, and being relegated to regular podiatry visits is not for everyone. Hammer toe surgery includes classic procedures that have been performed for decades and have stood the test of time, and new procedures developed more recently to improve results, reduce recurrences, and most importantly make life easier for the surgical patient.

When Bob came to us his toes were bent out of shape, red and sore, and had many painful corns. Bob was an executive at a big corporation and had to wear dress shoes most of the time. He had suffered for years and finally came in to see what could be done. After discussing all his options, Bob elected to have his hammer toes surgically fixed because he said he was fed up with his painful toes. We corrected one foot at a time, straightening multiple hammer toes on each, using the newest implants. He is now proud to show off his straight toes, and more importantly he has returned to his shoes pain-free.

How do I pick a surgeon?

How to choose a foot surgeon is discussed in detail in Chapter 20. All surgeons are not created equal, and selecting a skilled foot surgeon is crucial for success. Here let me remind you that board certification, routine performance of the procedure you are having done, recommendations from staff, positive word of mouth in your community, and happy patients are all good indicators of a skilled surgeon.

What are the surgical options for treating hammer toes?

Your foot surgeon will decide whether you are a good candidate for surgery and what procedure best fits your needs. In addition to an exam and x-rays, the surgeon takes many other factors into account, including your age, health, lifestyle, circulation, healing potentials, employment, the shoe you wish to wear postprocedure, time available for recovery, and goals. The goal of an eighty-year-old male with a hammer toe may be different from the goal a twenty-seven-year-old female.

Tenotomy

Tenotomies are performed to relieve flexible hammer toes. The procedure can be done through tiny incisions that heal quickly, making it the simplest hammer toe procedure to perform and also to recover from.

During a tenotomy, the surgeon releases the tight tendon responsible for the toe being in the hammer position. A Band-Aid or minimal dressing is all you need for aftercare, and recovery is speedy with a return to normal shoes often within a week.

This procedure is frequently performed on flexible hammer toes with painful corns on the tip of the toe. It is a popular option for seniors and diabetics, for whom the simplest procedure is the best option.

I wish a tenotomy could fix all hammer toes—it is so easy—but unfortunately, it only is appropriate for flexible hammer toes not rigid ones. Next up are the procedures used for the majority of hammer toe corrections.

Arthroplasty

An arthroplasty gives uniformly good results, eliminating painful hammer toes and returning toes to shoes comfortably. The procedure has been around forever because it is so successful and is the surgery of choice of many foot specialists. It is particularly useful for painful corns on fifth toes.

An arthroplasty realigns the toe by removing a small wedge of bone from the hammer toe. In essence, removing the protruding painful bump allows space for the toe to straighten and permanently resolves the hammer toe and painful corns.

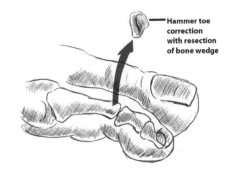

Hammer toe correction with resection of bone wedge

After the procedure, patients usually are placed in a surgical shoe with weight bearing allowed immediately. You can return to your own shoe, depending on the style, in anywhere from two to four weeks. Because the foot hangs down as we walk, it is not uncommon for swelling to occur. In most cases, in time the toe returns to normal size and is forever comfortable inside your shoes.

Arthrodesis

The difference between an arthroplasty and an arthrodesis is that in an arthroplasty bone is removed from the toe, and in an arthrodesis the toe is straightened by fusing the bone ends together.

Many podiatrists prefer an arthrodesis for correction, especially for the second and third toes. This is because the arthrodesis gives the toe a straighter appearance, has less chance of recurrence, usually heals with less swelling, and affords a long-lasting cosmetic result.

Recovery from the arthrodesis is similar to recovery from the arthroplasty—usually two to four weeks in a surgical shoe and a toe splint or bandage. Most surgeons choose to leave stitches in for about two weeks to ensure healing of the incision. During this period of recovery the surgical area is usually kept dry. Professional shower bags are often available from your surgeon to make bathing easier in the post-op period.

In the past, foot surgeons commonly used temporary pins to keep toes straight during healing. Unfortunately pins are inconvenient, uncomfortable, and unpopular with patients, so thankfully they are used only occasionally now.

Today, we have new implantable devices that eliminate the hassle of pins and provide better stability of the toe during healing and after. These small devices are made of biocompatible materials and don't need to be removed. Instead, they stay put, safely ensuring a permanent correction for hammer toes.

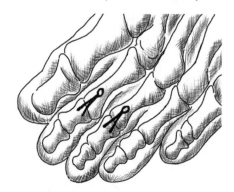

Hammer toe arthrodesis with internal fixation

Constant innovation continues to make foot surgery easier and more convenient for patients.

Will I have trouble walking with a fused toe?

Some patients are concerned that they will not be able to bend their toe after a surgical fusion and their gait will be affected. But to walk we actually need the foot to bend at the metatarsal joint, where the toe meets the foot. This joint is not affected by the toe surgery, and the fused toe supported by the implantable device makes a very good lever for moving you forward. So relax—a fused toe is no obstacle to walking, and it probably will even give you better stability.

Bone Spur Removal—Exostectomy

An exostectomy is a common procedure to remove a bone spur on a toe. Removing a bone spur is often done to treat corns between toes. This is a simple surgery to perform and also to heal from. The foot surgeon "shaves" off the spur, effectively eliminating the cause of the corn. The choice of procedure depends on location of the pain and what the surgeon feels is best for your long-term functional and cosmetic result, while limiting the chance of recurrence.

Let's Hammer It Out

So, in summation, if your toes hurt and are getting tender, twisted, bent, or buckled, it could be hammer time soon for you. Thankfully, with a skilled surgeon and new innovations, a result that combines pain relief and an appealing cosmetic outcome can return you to pain-free and fabulous feet!

Chapter 12

Morton's Neuroma: You've Got Nerve

W e usually associate a "pinched" nerve with a pain in the neck or back. But your feet also have nerves that can act up under pressure. A Morton's neuroma is a nerve in the ball of the foot that is feeling the crunch.

Bearing so much weight day in and day out, nerves in the bottom of the foot can become irritated. How people experience that irritation varies widely. Many complain of a sharp burning pain in the ball of their foot that may radiate into the toes. Some patients feel more of an ache, and others complain of numbness. Sometimes patients can link the discomfort to a specific activity or particular shoe, or they may find the pain to be completely unpredictable. Patients often report feeling as if they have something in their shoe. But when they take their shoe off to look, there is nothing in it.

Whatever way your nerve may signal to you it is not happy, a Morton's neuroma can make it difficult to get through your normal daily routine. Fortunately, podiatrists have options to give you and your nerve relief.

What is a neuroma?

It's a painful nerve in the ball of the foot. The nerve has grown, thickened, and scarred, becoming more of a bundle of nerves. The growth is benign and is a response to irritation. The nerves in the bottom of the foot normally look like very thick pieces of dental floss, white and glistening. If one of these nerves becomes traumatized over time, it thickens and looks almost like a small piece of chewing gum. This thickening of the nerve is medically termed *perineural fibrosis*. A doctor named Thomas George Morton was the first to describe the condition in the 1800s, and his name has been attached to it ever since.

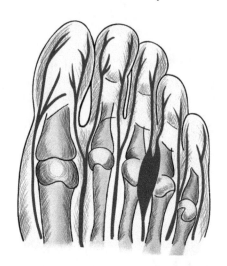

Neuromas usually occur in one of two spots on the foot. The most common place is between the third and fourth metatarsal bones, which are the long bones that span the arch and connect with the third and fourth toes. Patients usually feel pain on the ball of the foot often extending into toes three and four. The other common location is between the second and third metatarsal bones with pain also on the ball of the foot and extending to the second and third toes.

What irritated my nerve and made it painful?

There are many different causes of Morton's neuroma. You may never know for sure what caused your pinched foot nerve, but I've listed some common culprits below.

Heredity

The foot type you inherited may be to blame. Bone structure or alignment of the bones in the adult foot can contribute to developing neuromas. Some experts believe the metatarsal bones can be too close together, predisposing a person to pinching of the nerves between them.

Aging

Thinning of the skin on the bottom of the foot can contribute to a neuroma. As the fat padding and protective layers on the sole of the foot become thinner with age, the nerve endings become exposed and more vulnerable to increased trauma. Yet another benefit of growing older!

Sports

We often see Morton's neuromas in runners and other athletes, such as tennis players, who spend a lot of time on the balls of their feet.

Shoes

Wearing an uncomfortable shoe every day, such as a high heel or a pump, where the shoe directs pressure onto the ball of the foot, is a common cause of a Morton's neuroma. In general, shoes that are thin-soled, narrow, or high-heeled are likely to aggravate the condition. However, Morton's neuroma is also seen in men who have never donned a dress shoe or a high heel. Once a Morton's neuroma is present, shoes do make a difference because the wrong shoe can put pressure right on the painful nerve.

How do I know for sure I have a Morton's neuroma?

You will need to see a foot specialist to have your foot pain diagnosed. We mostly rely on an examination of the foot to diagnose a neuroma. Because nerves do not image on radiographs, x-rays aren't helpful in revealing a neuroma, but they can rule out other conditions that could be causing the pain, such as bone spurs or arthritis.

When a neuroma is suspected, your podiatrist may attempt to replicate the pain to determine if it is consistent with a neuroma. A specialist usually also checks for a *Mulder's sign*, which is a "clicking" sensation the patient feels when the forefoot is squeezed in a particular way. The click often reproduces the pain in the ball of the foot. In addition, your podiatrist might look for a *Sullivan's sign*, which is a spreading apart of toes in the area of the neuroma and often indicates the nerve is enlarging.

Because pain in the ball of the foot is not uncommon, foot specialists must consider other conditions. During the exam, we can rule out inflammation from the metatarsal bones (*capsulitis* or *metatarsalgia*), which can cause pain similar to a Morton's neuroma.

So based on a patient's description of symptoms, a clinical exam, pain, a Mulder's sign, a Sullivan's sign, and a high index of suspicion, a Morton's neuroma is often a relatively easy diagnosis for the specialist to make. When necessary, an MRI or ultrasound can be performed. Although not the gold standard for evaluating for neuroma, an ultrasound or MRI can be helpful to see if there is thickening of the nerve. In most cases, though, the clinical exam will provide enough information.

What are the treatment options?

Treatment options depend on how long the neuroma has been present and how painful the neuroma is. Some neuromas respond to conservative treatment. Others do not due to the amount of nerve damage. Because it is hard to determine how damaged the nerve is, most podiatrists recommend starting with conservative treatment. In about half the cases, the neuroma pain resolves.

What can I do at home to help relieve Morton's Neuroma?

The first line of action is to pay attention to your shoes. Here are some shoe tips to help take the pressure off that painful nerve.

Wear shoes in the house. Most of us can't wait to take our shoes off when we get home, but if you have a complaining nerve while barefoot, wear comfortable shoes inside to protect the bottom of the foot.

Get wider and larger shoes. Shift into a roomier shoe and make sure it has a wider width to allow more space for the toes and forefoot.

Try shoes with thick soles. Simply wearing a shoe that has a thick-soled bottom, like a running shoe or clog, can minimize continued irritation. This may take time, but the right shoes can diminish neuroma pain.

Carry an extra pair. Consider changing shoes when the neuroma starts to act up. Having a second pair to change into is helpful. This can shift the pressure off the neuroma and decrease discomfort.

Note the shoes that cause pain. If a shoe is predictably responsible for the pain, replace it. Experiment until you find a shoe that doesn't cause pain and gives your foot a break. This allows inflammation and swelling of the nerve to reduce over time.

Does massaging help?

Yes! When your nerve acts up, simply remove your shoe and massage the ball of your foot. It feels good and often the pain goes away.

Can I use topical creams?

Any type of topical anti-inflammatory rubbed into the foot can minimize pain and reduce inflammation. The relief may be temporary, but for an occasional nerve flare-up, it can be just the thing. For some anti-inflammatory options, check out those listed in Chapter 10 under Topicals.

What can the podiatrist do for me without surgery?

Orthotics and injections are both good choices for patients who have either mild cases of Morton's neuroma or prefer the least invasive form of treatment. Many foot specialists use a combination of paddings, orthotics, and injection therapy to treat the condition.

Orthotics

An orthotic is a shoe insert that is custom designed from casts taken of your foot. Orthotics for Morton's neuroma redistribute the pressure on the forefoot and spread the metatarsal bones slightly using protective pads under the ball of the foot. Although an orthotic may not work for all, it can do a wonderful job for many neuroma sufferers. And please note that orthotics can be designed for many styles and types of shoes, including women's dress shoes.

Injection Therapy

Injection therapy is the most common conservative treatment for Morton's neuroma. The injection is usually a combination of a local anesthetic mixed with a corticosteroid, which may reduce inflammation and scar tissue surrounding the neuroma. Although one injection can give relief, a series of injections can be more beneficial in providing a patient long-term success. Three seems to be the magic number to give more lasting results. It is difficult to predict which patients get relief from injection therapy; however, a good estimate is about half or more of the patients are relieved of pain.

Alcohol injections are another type of injection used to relieve a painful neuroma. Although it may sound like a martini mix is being used for treatment, this is not the case! An alcohol injection is a nonsteroidal injection of a medical-grade alcohol solution around the neuroma. The alcohol works to deaden the nerve endings to relieve sensitivity and pain. As with a corticosteroid, a series of alcohol injections is usually most beneficial and can give short- or long-term relief.

When should I consider surgery for my neuroma?

When conservative options no longer bring relief, it's time to consider surgery. It is not unusual, however, for a doctor to recommend surgery even before conservative therapy is attempted if the neuroma has been present for a significantly long time, and the patient does not want to attempt injection therapy or orthotics.

Regardless of which option you and your foot surgeon choose for an initial treatment plan, surgery is a common solution because conservative therapy is no guarantee of long-term pain relief. Just ask my patient Steven. Steven is an avid tennis player who can't go a week without playing. His neuroma had been painful off and on for years. He started with a series of injections, used custom sports orthotics, and wore wider shoes. This all helped, but every so often Steven came to the office for an injection to calm down his neuroma flare-up. He made it for many years, but recently came in and raised the white flag, asking for surgery and a permanent solution. His painful neuroma was removed, and he is now back on the tennis courts, happily roaming the baseline with no more foot faults!

How do I pick a surgeon?

How to choose a foot surgeon is discussed in detail in Chapter 20. All surgeons are not created equal, and selecting a skilled foot surgeon is crucial for success. Here let me remind you that board certification, routine performance of the procedure you are having done, recommendations from staff, positive word of mouth in your community, and happy patients are all good indicators of a skilled surgeon.

What procedure will my surgeon perform?

The most common procedure for a neuroma is a *neurectomy* in which the damaged portion of the nerve is removed, but there are other options, we will also discuss.

Neurectomy

The good news about having your Morton's neuroma removed is that this surgery is routinely performed and provides excellent results. Surgery is done on an outpatient basis, and because removing the neuroma is soft tissue surgery, with no bone involvement, healing is fairly easy for the majority of patients.

In most cases, the surgeon makes an incision on the top of the foot, which allows for postoperative weight bearing with a surgical shoe. The sutures are typically left in for about two weeks. Following suture removal, you can expect to return to normal activities including running, sports of all kinds, and even dress shoes, if that is your goal. This procedure is a clear winner!

Although relatively uncommon, there is a possible complication specific to neuroma surgery called a stump neuroma. This is a painful regrowth of a neuroma on the remaining end of the nerve after surgery. Should this occur, a second procedure is necessary to remove the stump neuroma and reposition the nerve to protect from this happening again.

Will my toes feel funny or be numb after surgery?

Many patients are concerned about how the foot may be affected after a nerve has been removed. It is important to note that this painful nerve is a sensory nerve and not a motor nerve. A sensory nerve conveys the feeling in the area, while a motor nerve controls function and movement. After Morton's neuroma surgery, normal motion and movement of the toes is maintained.

Because the nerve is a sensory nerve, sometimes there may be a small area of numbness, but this is not the kind that buzzes or becomes uncomfortable. If you touch the toe, you may not feel as much as you would touching the same toe on the other foot. In my thirty plus years of seeing patients after neuroma surgery, I can say it has been unusual for a patient to complain about numbness.

What are the other surgical options?

Skilled surgeons use techniques that they are competent performing and that have produced successful outcomes. Every surgeon has his or her own favorites to satisfy patients and, most importantly, relieve pain. Let's look at two alternatives to a traditional neurectomy.

Cryosurgery

In our practice, we also perform a procedure called cryosurgery to treat painful neuromas. Cryosurgery is a technique to freeze the neuroma rather than removing it. The procedure is minimally invasive and performed in the office. The foot specialist uses a local anesthetic and then makes a small incision in the foot. The cryosurgical probe is inserted and alternates between cycles that freeze and thaw the nerve. Although cryosurgery cannot guarantee elimination of neuroma pain permanently for all patients, many are extremely happy to have this option. This technique provides the benefit of a minimally invasive procedure and not having to remove the damaged nerve to give pain relief.

Melissa recently revisited our office, explaining that we had performed cryosurgery on her neuroma about seven years before. Her foot had felt great until recently. This recurrence of pain is not unusual. As opposed to removing the neuroma surgically, which is a permanent fix, cryosurgery may give the patient permanent pain relief, or there could be a return of symptoms down the road. Melissa said please "cryo" my neuroma again. We did, and she is hoping for another seven years of pain-free walking.

Podiatrists who perform cryosurgery are few and far between, so patients often travel long distances for treatment. We have patients come to us from all over the United States, from Canada, and from as far away as Russia to put a freeze on their painful neuromas.

Decompression Surgery

Unlike a neurectomy in which the nerve is removed, in this procedure, the nerve is "decompressed" by relieving the pressure on it. Releasing the ligament between the metatarsal bones that squeezes the nerve reduces the pressure on the neuroma, and thus relieves the pain.

The Nerve Ending

The pain from a Morton's neuroma can be quite debilitating, so see your podiatrist and start moving toward a solution. We have many options to help you quiet that nerve and let you get on with enjoying life. Remember, if you've gotta lot of nerve pain, we've gotta a lot of treatment options!

Chapter 13

Plantar Fasciitis:
The Real Deal about Painful Heels

I am often asked what is the most common painful condition we treat in our practice. My answer is always the same: plantar fasciitis. In our offices, not an hour goes by without seeing a patient for treatment of a painful heel. This condition has sidelined many a professional athlete—quarterbacks Peyton Manning, Eli Manning, and Drew Brees have all suffered through seasons of painful plantar fasciitis—and it can hobble us mere mortals too, driving out all thought except the pain from each and every step we take. Plantar fasciitis spares no one, from runners and athletes to moms, seniors, and everyone in between. If you see someone limping, there is a good chance they are being tormented by this condition. Over the last thirty years, plantar fasciitis seems to have risen to the status of epidemic or close to it. The good news is we have a multitude of treatments for this condition that resolve the pain. Consult your foot specialist about the best option for you, and don't let plantar fasciitis keep you out of the game.

How do I know if I have plantar fasciitis?

Have you ever woken up in the morning, swung your legs out of bed, stood up, and felt terrible heel pain? That's a classic sign of plantar fasciitis, which affects the thick band of connective tissue on the bottom of the foot. This band (the *plantar fascia)* supports four layers of muscles running from the heel through the arch of your foot to your toes. Pain is usually felt where the plantar fascia attaches to the bottom of the heel bone. When it becomes irritated and inflamed, you can count on the plantar fascia to speak out.

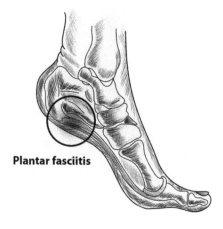

Plantar fasciitis

But shouldn't my heel feel better after a night's rest?

You would think so, but while you sleep or rest off your feet, the plantar fascia contracts and tightens. Just like any other body part might get a little stiff after you sit, so does this injured connective band. When you stand again, the contracted plantar fascia pulls tightly on the heel bone where it is attached and inflamed —"Ouch!"

My heel hurts all of the time, not just after resting.

You may feel the pain from an irritated plantar fascia some of the time (like on standing), or most of the time, or in severe cases, all of the time. The most common pain point is the heel, but the pain often extends into the arch. If untreated, the condition may worsen. Patients frequently come into our office limping because they have waited too long to seek treatment and now can't put any weight on the heel because of the pain.

Why did I get plantar fasciitis?

If you asked a dozen different doctors this question, you could get a dozen different answers, and each might be correct for a particular case. There are many causes of an inflamed plantar fascia. Let's look at what I consider the top five reasons for this type of heel pain. Of course, more than one factor can contribute to developing plantar fasciitis, and it is not uncommon for a combination of circumstances to add up to one terrible pain in the heel.

The Sports You Play

Stress, trauma, and overuse from participating in sports often irritate the plantar fascia. About 10 percent of all runners and athletes will suffer with heel pain at some point. Athletes find plantar fasciitis particularly frustrating to deal with for two reasons. Firstly, it can be difficult to treat while continuing to participate in a sport, and most runners and athletes can't stand to miss a game, a run, or an event. And secondly, this condition does not always heal as quickly as other injuries athletes frequently contend with.

The Extra Weight You Carry

I often tell my patients to pick up a ten-pound box and see how long it takes for their arms to tire out. It's usually only minutes before that box gets really heavy. When we put on weight, our feet have to carry those extra pounds around every day. They get tired and stressed, and the structures on the bottom of the feet responsible for holding it all up can get overworked and damaged. The good news is we can treat and cure plantar fasciitis regardless of body frame and current size, so you don't have to wait to reach the perfect number on the scale to get relief. Of course, I am an advocate for nutritious food choices and exercise. Any changes you make toward a healthier lifestyle are always appreciated by your feet!

The Shoes You Wear and the Surfaces You Work and Walk On

Your shoe choices matter when it comes to heel pain. Flip-flops, thin soled sandals, and slip-on flats offer minimal protection for the bottom of the feet, making the plantar fascia vulnerable to irritation and inflammation. Also, when your shoes get too old, the shock-absorbing materials wear out. More shock then goes into your foot and can lead to painful heels. If you have a job where you are on your feet all day, you are more likely to develop plantar fasciitis because the hard unyielding surfaces we work, shop, and walk on amplify the impact and stress on our feet.

The Foot Structure You Were Born With

There are three basic foot types: the flat foot, the normal arch, and the high-arched foot. Of course, there are millions of variations of each type, as no two feet are exactly the same, not even the two in a pair. In general, the flat foot is too flexible and tends to excessively roll inward with walking. This is called pronation, and it can contribute to stressing the plantar fascia and causing heel pain. A high arch can also lead to strain on the foot. High arches are usually rigid, which means they are poor shock absorbers. The extra wear and tear from taking a higher impact can irritate the heel.

The Stuff You Step On

I have seen countless patients who have stepped on something and triggered plantar fasciitis. Typical scenarios include stepping barefoot on a rock in the garden or driveway (known as a "stone bruise") and stepping on a child's toy in the house (I call this the "toy story"). Some parents have found their feet have a particular knack for finding Lego bricks in the dark. This kind of direct minor trauma can set off an inflammatory reaction that results in a painful episode of plantar fasciitis.

What can I do to self-treat my painful heel?

Self-treatment can be successful if begun early. First and foremost try to figure out what may have triggered your heel pain. Can you link your pain to a recent activity such as jogging, playing with the kids, shopping, visiting a museum, or even just a change in shoe style? If you suspect a connection, take a break from that activity until your heel feels better. You can also try the following recommendations.

Inspect and Evaluate Your Shoes

Are the soles of your shoes worn down or the cushioning deflated? Do you need a new pair? How long has it been since you went shoe shopping? Choose shoes with a firm thick sole. Women should avoid flat shoes and slip-ons. Believe it or not, a higher heel or wedge shoe is better for heel pain than a flat shoe, so change to shoes with an elevated heel. A clog can also be a good choice. A running sneaker usually has lots of shock absorption and cushioning, which can help too.

No Bare Feet

Not even in the house. Slip your feet directly into a shoe when you get out of bed. Continue to protect the heel until it gets better.

Ice It

Ice therapy is a great anti-inflammatory treatment and benefits are significant. It is easy to do, and you can fit it in around your schedule.

You can use an ice pack. I usually recommend a bag of frozen peas. The bag is flexible, covers a good amount of real estate on your foot, and is reusable without fuss or muss.

For those who are hearty, an ice bath is a good option. Put your painful foot into a bucket of water and add ice. An ice bath is mighty cold, but it's a great pain reliever. Professional athletes often soak their entire bodies in an ice bath to reduce aches and pains to get ready for the next game.

Another icy treatment is to put a bottle of water in the freezer and then roll the frozen water bottle back and forth over your heel and arch. This is a terrific way to combine deep massage and cold therapy.

Try Topical Anti-inflammatories

Along with ice, any over-the-counter topical anti-inflammatory agent can offer pain relief and swelling reduction. For an expanded list of anti-inflammatories, see Topicals in Chapter 10.

Try Oral Anti-inflammatories

Over-the-counter medications such as Advil or Aleve can afford some pain relief to help get through the day.

Stretch

Keeping your calf muscles stretched is important for resolving heel pain. The more you stretch the better. The two best stretches are the wall stretch and the stair stretch.

The *wall stretch* is a classic stretch runners have used for decades. Place both hands on a wall with your heel flat on the floor and simply lean in and feel the stretch in your calf muscle. Do this stretch both with your knee straight and then bent to most effectively stretch all the muscles in your calf. Stretching should not cause pain. Just lean until you feel the stretch and hold it for a few

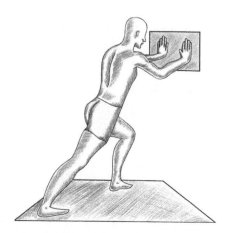

seconds. Repeat a number of times. Then repeat daily and often. Just think of how a cat stretches throughout the day, and you get the idea.

To try the *stair stretch*, stand on a stair and let your heel hang backward off the end of the stair as if it were reaching to the stair below. Two to three seconds is good, then lift up your heel and relax. Repeat about ten times. Hold onto the railing for balance as necessary. Again, just feel the stretch and back off if you feel pain.

Use Inserts

In general, any additional cushioning or support under your heel and foot can reduce pain and make walking more comfortable. Prefabricated arch supports and heel cups are the first line of therapy for heel pain. Custom orthotics are reviewed later in the chapter under Supporting the Plantar Fascia.

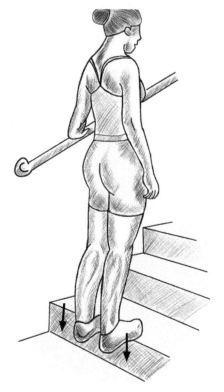

When should I see a podiatrist about my heel pain?

If you have attempted any, many, or none of the above self-treatments, and your heel pain persists, the podiatrist is your next stop. In general, any time you have pain failing to resolve after one or two weeks, it is appropriate to schedule an appointment. Also, the longer you have heel pain, the harder it may become to eliminate it on your own.

What will the podiatrist do at my appointment?

When I see a patient with heel pain, my first task is to make a differential diagnosis. This means there are several conditions that could be causing the pain, and it must be determined which one is behind the symptoms. Plantar fasciitis is by far the most common cause of heel pain, but there are others that can lead to pain in the same location. These include a stress fracture, nerve entrapments such as *tarsal tunnel syndrome* and *Baxter's nerve entrapment*, heel bursitis, a ruptured plantar fascia, bone cysts in the heel bone, and soft tissue masses in the heel area.

To determine your primary condition, your podiatrist will review your history, examine your foot, and probably do some additional testing.

What tests will the podiatrist order?

Although your podiatrist may have a high level of confidence in a diagnosis from your history and the location and quality of your pain, most foot specialists perform some type of imaging study. Usually podiatrists take x-rays first, which can reveal a heel spur (an indicator of plantar fasciitis) and possibly a stress fracture or a bone cyst if present.

What x-rays do not show is the plantar fascia itself, which is a soft tissue structure not visible on radiographs. So why take the x-rays? Because it is important to rule out or discover these other conditions. Many podiatrists then use ultrasound imaging—an excellent diagnostic tool—to view the plantar fascia, determine how inflamed or injured it is, and confirm a diagnosis of plantar fasciitis.

What is a heel spur?

Spurs are bony calcium deposits that develop in response to stress. Remember the plantar fascia is attached to the heel, so when this connective band tightens, it pulls and irritates from its attachment point on the heel bone. In response to this stress, the heel slowly forms more bone—a heel spur—leaving patients with an extra bony growth on the bottom of their heel.

If I have a spur, shouldn't it be removed?

No, not usually. Unfortunately, too much emphasis is placed on whether a heel spur is present. In most cases, the spur is not the source of the pain. This was not understood years ago when everyone thought the spur was the problem and that the spur had to be removed to relieve heel pain. Over time, surgeons realized the painful part of the condition was not the spur, but the inflamed and injured fascia that pulls on the spur. This was a big "Aha moment."

I often describe the relationship of the plantar fascia to the heel bone with this analogy: if you pull on your hair, your scalp hurts; but to eliminate the pain, you don't remove the scalp, you just stop pulling on it. This understanding came too late for Joltin' Joe DiMaggio whose baseball career was ruined by heel pain and the subsequent surgery to remove the bone spur. Back then doctors only had x-rays for diagnosis, and the surgery was relatively primitive.

Since then, innovative treatments and procedures have been developed to treat chronic heel pain. If surgery is ever necessary, the plantar fascia can simply be released from its attachment point to the heel where it is causing the pain. Then the fascia no longer tugs on the heel, and patients are cured of heel pain without the spur being removed. Today the spur has finally been relegated to an incidental finding.

But we have gotten ahead of ourselves by talking about surgery. Let's return to conservative treatment, which cures many cases of plantar fasciitis without the patient ever needing to have surgery.

How will the doctor treat my plantar fasciitis?

After the diagnosis of plantar fasciitis is confirmed, a foot doctor usually starts a conservative care plan. The goal of treatment in our practice is simple: to relieve your pain and return you to normal activities. We accomplish this by focusing on decreasing inflammation, stretching tight structures, and supporting the foot. Often we start working on all three at once.

Decreasing Inflammation

Although there are many options to reduce internal inflammation, corticosteroid injection is a strong anti-inflammatory and works quickly. When plantar fasciitis pain is severe, most patients appreciate fast and effective pain relief.

An important benefit of an injection is placement of the medicine exactly where it is needed. Many podiatrists use ultrasound-guided injections, which allow for precise placement of the corticosteroid in the spot that is most inflamed. Ultrasound can also be used to monitor progress and determine if further anti-inflammatory treatments are needed.

Although it is natural for some to have a fear of injections, most patients are happy to have "braved" a shot because of the pain relief received. The other good news is that only a small amount of cortisone is needed to heal the plantar fasciitis, reducing concern about medication side effects. You can expect one to three injections, depending on the severity of the pain.

Podiatrists have additional treatment options to reduce the inflammation associated with an irritated or damaged plantar fascia. Nonsteroidal anti-inflammatories (NSAIDs) are commonly recommended and effective. Your doctor may choose a prescription-strength NSAID for you. Like all prescription medications, side effects are possible, most commonly stomach issues. Physical therapy, daily icing, and rest also can help to quiet heel pain.

Stretching Using a Night Splint

Because a major cause of plantar fasciitis is a tightening and contracting of the plantar fascia, stretching becomes a most important part of your treatment plan. In addition to recommending the calf stretches discussed in the self-treatment section, many foot specialists dispense or prescribe a *plantar fascial night splint* to wear at bedtime. This has proven to be a mainstay to help patients eliminate morning pain, and studies have confirmed it is an excellent conservative treatment.

Although sleeping with a brace on your foot and leg can be challenging at first, most patients do surprisingly well. This is a simple and highly effective way to stretch your calf muscles and plantar fascia and relieve morning pain.

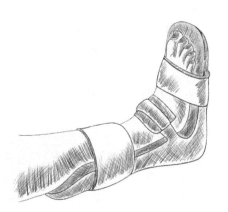

Supporting Your Plantar Fascia

Your foot specialist can supply or recommend appropriate supportive devices to ensure you do not continue to strain an injured plantar fascia. It is difficult to truly rest a foot, so it becomes vital to add support to not compromise healing. Commonly used techniques include tapings and strappings, premade plantar fascial straps, CAM walker boots, over-the-counter arch supports, and custom orthotics.

Your foot will appreciate any and all support; however, most podiatrists recommend a custom orthotic because of the long-term benefits for managing plantar fasciitis. Orthotics made from casts of your feet support the plantar fascia, relieve chronic strain, and minimize recurrence.

What happens if the pain doesn't go away?

In our office, we monitor the most painful cases of plantar fasciitis regularly until there is significant relief from the pain. We continue to see our patients until the pain is at a level of *zero*. That is the goal, and you should expect complete pain relief with treatment and time. Plantar fasciitis unresponsive to treatment for longer than six months is referred to as chronic. But don't despair, we have several treatment options for stubborn heel pain.

RPT: Radial Pulse Therapy:

RPT is a state-of-the-art non-surgical treatment to relieve painful plantar fasciitis. RPT uses targeted radial pulses, a form of mechanical energy, and delivers treatment into previously difficult to reach injured tissue areas. RPT is performed without need for local anesthesia and is usually five treatments performed over 3-5 weeks. Each treatment delivers 3200 "shocks" to the area in about 5 minutes. There are usually no limitations on activity following RPT treatment.

ESWT: Extra Corporeal Shock Wave Therapy:

ESWT is similar to RPT in that it delivers targeted mechanical energy into the deep tissue layers. ESWT provides what is known as "high energy" shock waves, similar to how lithotripsy is used to treat kidney stones. ESWT is a one-time treatment procedure requiring local anesthesia. The intense delivery of shock wave energy into the area triggers the injured plantar fascia to return to normal usually over 4-12 weeks post treatment. Patients are usually placed in a walking boot for a few weeks to allow for healing.

Our practice has been fortunate to employ these technologies for many years. RPT and ESWT are the go-to conservative treatments of choice for many podiatrists and their patients because of the stellar results afforded non-surgically. Both provide excellent long-term relief. Over the past few years RPT, has proven to be more popular of the two choices because of the ease of treatment and limited after-care needed.

Platelet-Rich Plasma Injections

These injections have gained popularity in the athletic community. Numerous professional athletes have tried platelet-rich plasma injections (PRP) for plantar fasciitis and other injuries. Using PRP is a simple procedure. First, a vial of your blood is drawn, and then spun down in a centrifuge to isolate the platelets. Your "platelet-rich" blood is then injected back into your plantar fascia. The theory is platelet-rich blood has great healing potentials. PRP injection is a conservative treatment and carries minimal risk. Success rates vary, and in my experience are not nearly as uniform as those from using RPT or ESWT.

Cryosurgery

Cryosurgery is a technique that freezes the plantar fascia in an attempt to cure the pain. Cryosurgery is minimally invasive, the plantar fascia is left intact, there is minimal postprocedure discomfort, and it provides a high success rate. Although an effective technique, cryosurgical machines are few and far between, so it may be difficult to locate a specialist who performs cryosurgery.

Plantar Fascial Release

If surgery becomes necessary, plantar facial release is the go-to option. Most surgeons perform the procedure through a fairly small incision on the inside of the heel. By releasing the plantar fascia from the attachment point, it is no longer able to excessively pull on the heel bone, thus eliminating the pain. The tension on the plantar fascia is relieved. Remember our hair pulling analogy? If the hair is no longer pulling on the scalp, the scalp doesn't hurt.

In many cases, it is only necessary to release a part of the plantar fascia. It is important to note that nothing is removed during surgery, and the plantar fascia remains in your foot and still serves a function. It just won't cause any more pain. We expect our surgical patients to be completely relieved of pain and return to all preoperative activities.

Why does my child have heel pain?

Heel pain in children ages eight to fourteen is usually attributed to the growth plate. In this age range, the heel bone is still growing, and the growth plate remains open. Stress, trauma, foot type, sports, and other activities can all put a strain on the growth plate resulting in significant pain.

It is important for parents to understand this does not affect the growth of the bone. It can, however, cause a lot of discomfort. It is also important to understand this is a condition, not a disease. I usually refer to this as *apophysitis* and not by the common term *Sever's disease*, which sounds more than a bit scary.

Apophysitis frequently occurs in children who participate in sports. The foot becomes too painful to run on, and the kids are often seen limping either during or after activities. I diagnosed Kristy, a twelve-year-old dancer, with apophysitis after she had been putting in extra hours preparing for a performance. The bottom and both sides of her heel were painful, but not swollen or red. Homecare included resting (no jumping, no gym), icing, stretching, a heel lift, and wearing a strap during the day and a splint at night. I also fitted her for orthotics. Kristy was back dancing in less than four weeks.

Children either with high arched feet or excessively flat feet that pronate (roll in) and children who are overweight are especially vulnerable to this condition. Treatments include resting from sports, heel lifts, icing, anti-inflammatories, orthotics, and immobilization if necessary. If your child has heel pain, consult with your podiatrist to determine the cause and best treatment to help quickly resolve the pain.

Put your heel pain behind you!

Plantar fasciitis is one of the most common, painful problems affecting the foot and can suddenly stop life in its tracks. Now that you know the real deal on heel pain, you no longer have to suffer. Foot specialists treat plantar fasciitis on a daily basis, and we are happy to report if you have plantar fasciitis, you can become one of the many who one day say, "I *had* plantar fasciitis."

Chapter 14

The Achilles:
A Hero of a Tendon

You have probably heard of the Greek warrior Achilles, who had only one vulnerable spot, the tendon at the back of the heel. His mother, a sea nymph, dipped him as a newborn in the magical River Styx, and everywhere the water touched the baby he became protected from harm. But his mother held him just above his heel as she lowered him into the water, and this became his secret weakness. No one could defeat the magnificent warrior, who seemed indestructible as a god, until eventually an arrow hit the mark, and Achilles died, pierced in the tendon where his mother's fingers had held him.

The tendon that we can all feel running from the back of the heel up our lower leg is the only part of our body that bears a hero's name. It is deserved. The Achilles is the thickest tendon in the body. It has to be big and strong because it does a difficult task. It lifts our heel from the ground each time we take a step—that's thousands of times a day. Quite a workload! But that heavy lifting also makes the Achilles tendon vulnerable. We can overwork it and not listen when it tells us to rest. Eventually it can become damaged and painful.

If this tendon has become your weak spot, stiff and sore, painful, or visibly inflamed, read on. You may have Achilles tendonitis, and there are many treatment options to help your hero of a tendon recover its powers. Or you may have a different variety of Achilles problem, and we'll discuss some of those as well.

Who is likely to get Achilles tendonitis?

The Achilles acts up when it is overstressed. Athletes often suffer from Achilles tendonitis, but this condition can also plague weekend warriors, power shoppers, vacationers, senior citizens, and children—just about anyone who suddenly asks their tendon to do more than it is accustomed to.

Here are two examples of recently treated patients with tender tendons: Erin, a twenty-five-year-old runner who was preparing for a 10K race, and Gordon, a fifty-six-year-old who had just returned from a two-week tour of Italy. Their stories have a common theme—overuse, too much too soon, and more activity than normal for that individual. Both patients had asked their Achilles to work harder and longer than it was used to and ended up in pain. If you have been engaging in activity that is unusual for you and find your Achilles is aching, see a podiatrist. You may need some help healing your new weak spot.

How do I avoid getting Achilles tendonitis?

Tendonitis is the result of stress. The body can adjust to stress without becoming injured if given enough time and preparation. For an athlete, this means planned training that builds up slowly and carefully to events. (See Chapter 5, "Fun and Games: Prevent, Prepare, and Play Like a Pro," for more about preventing sports injuries.) The advice is the same for anyone who has an activity coming up that is unusual for their body, whether that is a vacation at Disney World or a charity walk-a-thon, a hiking trip with your college buddies or a weekend shopping with your best friend. Your body can take on added challenges, if you are prepared.

How do I know if I have Achilles tendonitis?

Pain around or above the back of the heel is the big indicator. Podiatrists diagnose Achilles tendonitis from reported symptoms and an exam. We stage it too. The condition can be mild, moderate, or severe. Let's discuss each stage in turn.

Mild

The early stage of Achilles tendonitis is marked by as a combination of stiffness and pain. The tendon is often stiff in the morning or after sitting. After the tendon loosens up, walking is often pain-free; however, it may become painful with extended walking. By the end of the day, the tendon is usually tight and sore. The tendon may not look swollen or inflamed and may still appear similar to the tendon of the other foot. You may feel pain when you squeeze the tendon between your fingers.

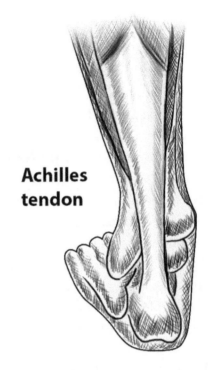

Achilles tendon

Moderate

This stage is what most refer to as plain old Achilles tendonitis, probably because the medical term, *paratenonitis*, is too hard to pronounce. This stage certainly is not too hard to recognize. The tendon is visibly swollen and much more painful than in the early stage. This is because the outer layer of the tendon, actually a sheath around the tendon called the *paratenon*, is now affected. Performing in sports or even walking normally becomes difficult because of increased pain and swelling.

Severe

In this advanced stage, sufferers will note a significant change in the tendon. It appears to be thickened and even bulbous. Whereas moderate Achilles tendonitis affects the outer layer of the tendon, in this stage, known as *tendonosis*, there is damage to the actual tendon itself. Tendonosis is similar to a scar that leaves the skin

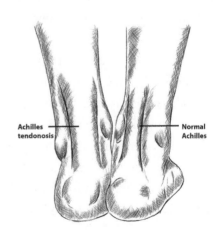

Achilles tendonosis · Normal Achilles

abnormally thick or raised. As the Achilles tendon and tendon fibers become increasingly damaged, the reaction of the tendon is to thicken or scar. This may be a defense mechanism to prevent the tendon from tearing completely. An Achilles tendonosis is hard to heal, and for some the tendon stays permanently thickened and painful.

When should I see a podiatrist?

Don't wait! When you feel that pain in the tendon, make an appointment. All three stages of tendon stress described above—mild, moderate, and severe—are commonly referred to as Achilles tendonitis. However, their symptoms, as we have noted, are not the same, and healing success rates differ as well. The earliest stage of Achilles tendonitis is fairly easy to get back to normal, while the later-stage tendonosis, can be quite debilitating and difficult to heal or improve. This is why professional evaluation of your particular Achilles injury is so important. The sooner the area is evaluated and treated, the better.

What can I do at home to treat my tendonitis?

Home treatment of early-stage tendonitis includes the usual therapies for injuries. In this case, we use the PRICE method: Protect, Rest, Ice, Cut Back, and Elevate.

Protect your Achilles from further injury. A simple tendonitis can advance to a long-term painful tendonosis. We live with the consequences of our actions. If we don't take that week or two to rest, it could mean months to heal. My favorite two-letter word sentence applies: "If it is to be, it is up to me." Take time to heal right the first time. Achilles injuries can become chronically painful, so it is best to get professional guidance and treat this injury with respect.

Rest is always the key to success, the more the better. Fewer steps reduce the workload on the tendon. The less work for the tendon, the quicker it heals.

*Ice i*s a primary anti-inflammatory treatment. A flexible ice pack that wraps around the entire tendon works best. For the hearty, the perfect treatment is to soak in an ice-water bath up to the midcalf. Another technique is ice massage. Fill a paper cup with water and freeze. Massage the tendon with the cup, and then use your fingers to massage the painful tendon. Massaging an Achilles tendonitis is a popular way to help speed healing.

Cut back on activities. For athletes, decreasing your workouts, your speed, and all training routines is a must. Full participation risks further injury, delayed healing, and rupture of the tendon. The rule of thumb with Achilles injuries is if it hurts, don't do it. Simple as that. With this injury it is best not to push through pain.

Elevate in this context means to elevate the heel in the shoe. Remember the job of the tendon is to lift the heel up when walking. If the heel is raised with a heel lift or an elevated shoe, it makes the job easier on the tendon. It puts "slack in the line" and relieves pressure on the injured tendon. Flat shoes are the worst to wear with an Achilles injury. Wedged shoes, cowboy boots, or placing a heel lift at least a quarter-inch thick in the shoe are all good options. This is one instance when your podiatrist might actually recommend a higher-heeled shoe.

What treatment options can a podiatrist offer?

The most important task of your foot specialist is to accurately diagnose your injury and guide you through the fastest and best course of treatment. PRICE is always the baseline for treatment. In addition, here are more options to help heal an injured Achilles.

NSAIDs: Nonsteroidal Anti-inflammatories

NSAIDs are a commonly used and effective treatment for Achilles tendonitis. Your doctor may prescribe a prescription-strength medication to decrease inflammation. Like all prescription medications, side effects are possible, most commonly stomach issues.

Topical Anti-inflammatories

Both prescription and over-the-counter topical medications are used for this condition. Topical medications are placed directly on the injured area. See the list of anti-inflammatories given in Chapter 10 under Topicals for some options.

Night Splints

Gentle stretching of the tendon can be helpful, while aggressive stretching could cause additional pain. Utilizing a special night splint provides gentle stretching for the tendon and muscles in the back of the leg. The night splint is effective at eliminating morning stiffness and helps with rehabilitation of the tendon. Stretching should be pain-free or minimally uncomfortable.

Physical Therapy (PT)

Physical therapy is recommended for sufferers of Achilles tendonitis. Different techniques, including ultrasound, electrical stimulation, and cold laser therapy, are beneficial to enhance healing the tendon. The initial goal of PT is to reduce inflammation and pain. Once accomplished, rehabilitation and strengthening of the tendon are the next priorities.

Eccentric (Pronounced "E-centric") Stretching

This is a special stretching technique that has been shown to be effective in rehabilitation and strengthening of the Achilles tendon, but you don't have to be an eccentric to do it. This form of stretching can help the tendon fibers remodel, strengthen, and heal. It is different from the standard stretching. An example of an eccentric stretch is to stand on a step and carefully let the injured heel stretch downward toward the stair below, and then using both feet, pull the heels up. Repeat this cycle.

Important Note Regarding Cortisone Injections

It is as important to know what *not* to do, as it is what to do, when being treated for this injury. Cortisone injections fall into the "what not to do" category. Although cortisone injections offer effective treatment for many injuries, it is not advised for your Achilles. Injecting cortisone in or around your Achilles tendon places your tendon at increased risk of tendon rupture.

Orthotics

Custom orthotic inserts are a staple of long-term treatment for Achilles tendonitis. Orthotics offer the benefit of not only elevating the heel but also providing what is called *triplane correction.* One of the related causes of Achilles tendonitis is the "whipping" motion of the tendon when excessive pronation is present. Minimizing pronation, elevating the heel, and keeping the foot moving straight ahead without turning too far in or out, relieves stress on the Achilles.

Radial Pulse Therapy (RPT) & Extracorporeal Shock Wave Therapy (ESWT)

RPT and ESWT are noninvasive procedure used to help heal chronic Achilles tendonitis unresponsive to the usual treatments. It is based on technology called *lithotripsy* that breaks up kidney stones and is also used for treating plantar fasciitis and tennis elbow. RPT and ESWT deliver focused energy, or shockwaves, to the tendon, which stimulates healing. High-energy ESWT is a one-time treatment requiring local anesthesia. RPT requires no anesthesia and patients usually require five treatments for maximal results. See also under the treatment for plantar fasciitis in chapter 13.

Platelet-Rich Plasma (PRP) Injections

These injections are another technique to help heal chronic painful Achilles tendonitis that is not responsive to conservative treatment. The procedure uses a patient's own blood to stimulate healing. First, a vial of the patient's blood is put into a centrifuge and spun-down, separating the platelet-rich plasma that contains what is known as *human growth factors*. The platelet-rich plasma is then injected into the injured area of the tendon. This treatment has become popular, especially for professional athletes, who want to attempt quicker healing of the tendon. It's also used to speed healing of plantar fasciitis (See Chapter 13, "Plantar Fasciitis: The Real Deal about Heel Pain").

Immobilization

Sometimes an effective treatment is to wear a CAM walker boot or a cast to protect and rest the tendon. This is especially helpful for those in severe pain who are not responding to conservative treatments. Anywhere from three to six weeks of immobilization can be effective.

MRI Imaging

An MRI is not a treatment; however, it is often helpful in providing more exact diagnosis of the injury, and thus can help your doctor select the most effective treatment plan for you. Because the Achilles tendon is not seen on x-rays, the best way to visualize the tendon is through MRI. An MRI readily shows inflammation and can reveal if there is a partial or complete tear of the tendon. Often a small partial tear is a reason the tendon does not respond to treatment. An ultrasound is another imaging technique that can be helpful to visualize injury to the Achilles tendon.

Surgery for Achilles Tendonitis and Achilles Tendonosis

Surgery is a last resort for this condition; however, it is an option for those who have tried everything without results. At least six months or more of conservative therapy is recommended before surgery is considered. Surgery on the tendon removes scar tissue, damaged tendon fibers, and sutures the weakened portion of the tendon. If necessary, a tendon graft is used to secure and strengthen the tendon. Rehabilitation takes time. It can be months before you resume normal activities, but surgery does resolve the chronic pain for most.

How do I pick a surgeon?

How to choose a foot surgeon is discussed in detail in Chapter 20. All surgeons are not created equal, and selecting a skilled foot surgeon is crucial for success. Here let me remind you that board certification, routine performance of the procedure you are having done, recommendations from staff, positive word of mouth in your community, and happy patients are all good indicators of a skilled surgeon.

What about when an Achilles tendon ruptures?

A complete tear of the Achilles tendon is not uncommon. The rupture is usually sudden and painful. For many, it is an injury that occurs on the athletic field.

A host of famous athletes have suffered this difficult, career-threatening condition. Basketball player Kobe Bryant, soccer player David Beckham, and football quarterback Dan Marino all have suffered torn Achilles tendons. Ironically, Brad Pitt, who played the role of Achilles in the movie *Troy*, also is said to have injured his Achilles during the filming of the movie.

The diagnosis of a rupture is immediate and confirmed by MRI. Treatment is either surgery or casting. Because both treatments can be successful, it is for the surgeon and patient to decide which course is best. Healing and rehabilitation take months. Ruptured tendons can be difficult to return to as good as new and require intensive therapy to get back to preinjury status.

Are there other common problems involving the Achilles?

A variety of other conditions can develop that involve the Achilles tendon. As always, having a podiatrist make a diagnosis of any pain affecting the tendon is key to finding the speediest path to recovery

Why do I have pain in the back of my heel?

That pain could indicate you have *insertional tendonitis* and *retro-calcaneal bone spurs*. Bear with me! It's less complicated than it sounds. The Achilles tendon extends from the muscles in the back of the leg to the heel and attaches to the entire back portion of the heel bone, the calcaneus. This attachment point, called the insertion, can become painful for many reasons, but the most common is a tight Achilles tendon that is pulling too strongly—insertional tendoniti*s*. The heel bone becomes irritated and reacts by growing a bone spur, a retro-calcaneal bone spur to be exact. X-rays are used to diagnose the spur, but the standard treatments for tendonitis

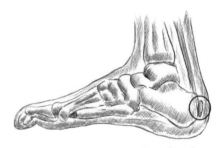

Retrocalcaneal spur

discussed earlier in the chapter usually resolve the pain. If the pain does not improve, the spur may need to be removed surgically.

What is that bump that sticks out on the back of my heel?

A bony enlargement on the back of the heel bone may be a *Haglund's deformity*. It is often called a "pump bump" because it becomes painful and irritated from women's dress shoes, although men can develop these bumps as well. It might seem that the Achilles is involved in this problem, but in most cases, the Achilles tendon is not the cause of the bone enlargement.

Changing shoes that irritate the bump is the simplest solution, but if a new shoe choice doesn't bring relief, the bump may need to be removed. Fortunately, this surgery can usually be done without any disruption to the Achilles tendon.

Keep Achilles Strong

Whether you are a godlike Greek warrior or just an ordinary mortal, your Achilles tendon plays a vital role in your daily life. If your Achilles starts to bother you, seek professional help from your foot and ankle specialist. This is one injury that requires professional evaluation, accurate diagnosis, and early treatment, to help ensure you are not left with your own "Achilles' heel."

Chapter 15

Ankles:
The Twists and Turns

Your ankle and foot are a dynamic duo. Working together they help you stand, balance, walk, and run. Any injury to the ankle weakens this partnership, affects your mobility, and can keep you from getting where you need to go. Just one serious ankle injury may set you up for a future of many twists and turns.

Think of your ankle as a busy hub where multiple parts meet, connect, and pass through. Three bones come together to form the ankle joint: two leg bones (the tibia and fibular) and one foot bone (the talus). They are held together by a series of ligaments that run along both sides and in front and back of the ankle. Ten different tendons pass by the ankle to perform their duties in the foot, not to mention the nerves that also course through the area.

With all these components, there are many possibilities for something in

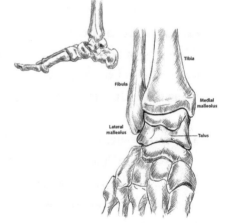

your ankle going awry. So often it is a simple trip or slip that causes ankles to give way and damage to be done to bones, ligaments, cartilage, or tendons. But with timely attention and care, most ankle problems can be righted. And the ankle can return to playing its part in helping you stay up and at 'em.

I twisted my ankle—when should I see a doctor?

Watch for swelling and changes in color to black, blue, and purple; these usually indicate a more serious injury. Pain is also a guide. The more pain you feel, generally the more extensive the damage. So, if your ankle is swollen and screaming, go to an emergency room or specialist's office—pronto.

How will my ankle injury be diagnosed?

An urgent care facility or emergency room will rely on x-rays. If your ankle is fractured, the injury will be obvious on an x-ray, and treatment started immediately. The fracture is usually put in a cast for four to six weeks, followed by rehabilitation. In most cases, the cast and therapy allow broken ankles to heal as good as new. If severely broken, dislocated, or out of alignment, the ankle fracture may need surgical repair.

If x-rays of your ankle do not reveal a fracture, the diagnosis is often a sprain. You will be given a temporary ankle wrap (for compression and stability) with standard instructions to rest, ice, and follow up with a specialist for further evaluation to ensure proper healing.

What can I do at home to treat a sprained ankle?

If the sprain appears minor with limited swelling or bruising, or you have been sent home from the ER with a sprain diagnosis, you may begin home treatment with RICE (Rest, Ice, Compression, Elevation).

- *Rest*: Sometimes the hardest thing to do and also the most important. If an activity hurts, cease and desist!
- *Ice:* The more the better. At least fifteen minutes of every waking hour for the first two to three days.
- *Compression:* Depending on the severity of the ankle injury, use a compression bandage or an ankle brace to protect the ankle and

minimize pain and swelling. Wear until all swelling and pain is resolved or until your specialist says you can safely remove it.

- *Elevate:* Keep your foot elevated above your heart to minimize swelling and pain.

Remember, it is essential to follow up with a specialist if recommended by the emergency care doctor, or if your pain and symptoms do not improve quickly.

A sprained ankle is not a big deal, right?

Have you heard the old saying "A sprain can be worse than a break"? Well, it's true and for the following reason: a broken ankle gets immediate diagnosis and treatment, while a sprain is often minimized, treatment neglected, and damaged ligaments left weakened. Many patients hear the words "not broken," and then think the injury is not so serious. They often fail to follow up with a specialist, skip rehabilitation of the ankle, and leave ligaments stretched—or worse, torn—and vulnerable to further injury and instability.

How do I know if my sprain is a serious one?

Ankle sprains are graded in stages. Stage 1 is mild with stretching of ligaments. Stage 2 is moderate with partial tearing of one or more ligaments. Stage 3 is severe with complete rupture of one or more ligaments.

Unfortunately, standard x-rays do not show ligaments, so doctors can't use them to see stretching, partial tears, or ruptures. That's why a follow-up visit to a foot specialist is important after an ankle injury.

What will my foot specialist do?

First and most importantly, your podiatrist will perform a complete examination to determine integrity of the ankle, the ligaments, and surrounding structures that are often injured when an ankle is sprained. Then a decision will be made as to whether further imaging is necessary, the length of time needed for immobilization, when full weight bearing can begin, and referral for physical therapy if necessary.

Our patient Peter had just this kind of evaluation. A nineteen-year-old cross country runner, Peter came into our office referred by the local hospital's ER. During a training run, he had stepped on a tree root and severely twisted his ankle. He said it swelled up like a balloon immediately, and he couldn't put any weight on it. X-rays did not show a fracture, but he was in severe pain, his ankle had all the pretty colors of the rainbow, and he could barely move it.

In our office, we performed special stress x-rays and determined Peter had damaged but not completely ruptured the ligaments on the outside of his ankle. His ankle was first placed in a special compression bandage to get the swelling down with limited weight bearing and then placed in a CAM walker boot to protect the ankle. After one week, the bandage was removed and Peter was sent to physical therapy where they performed functional rehabilitation on his ankle.

What does ankle rehabilitation entail?

In the past, most ankle injuries were treated with long periods of immobilization and no weight bearing. Now the standard is early rehabilitation through active therapy. The goals of PT are to

- reduce pain and inflammation as quickly as possible,
- improve range of motion to preinjury levels,
- rehabilitate ligaments,
- strengthen the ankle and surrounding muscles and tendons,
- provide balance training, and
- return patients to their normal activities, including sports, without further injury risk.

It is essential for the ligaments to heal to ensure no residual chronic weakness that leads to recurrent spraining.

During his rehabilitation, Peter checked in at our office every couple of weeks, so we could monitor his progress. Because of the early intervention and therapy, Peter was able to get back to competitive running wearing a supportive ankle brace in just four weeks. His story is a great example of not neglecting treatment for sprains.

I have repeatedly sprained my ankle, what's going on?

Ligaments are like rubber bands. They work fine when tight and strong. But if you suffer either a severe sprain or a series of minor sprains, the ligaments can become so stretched, weakened, or torn, that they no longer firmly hold the foot and ankle bones together. Eventually, the ankle becomes unstable, resulting in chronic sprains and pains.

That's what happened to Caitlyn, who came to our office complaining that for years her ankle had felt weak and unstable. She was thirty-five and had been a serious gymnast when she was younger. She had started competing at the age of five and was top in her high school district, often competing at the national level. Through the years of practices and meets, there were more than a few dismounts and tumbles that had bent her ankle in ways she would rather not remember. Yes, she missed some time here and there from her ankle sprains, but she would be back at the gym as soon as she possibly could with tape and braces holding her ankle together.

Though Caitlyn had not competed in over a decade, when she came to see us, her ankles were more vulnerable than ever. She could not wear dress shoes with any heel, and even with simple walking her ankles could just give out. We evaluated Caitlyn's ankles and found they were significantly unstable and loose. The joint was fine on x-rays; however, an MRI showed complete ruptures of two of her ankle ligaments. Physical therapy did not improve her status, so Caitlyn eventually had her ligaments repaired to strengthen and "tighten up" her ankle.

How are torn ligaments repaired?

If like Caitlyn, you end up with chronic ankle instability and pain, the good news is that new procedures are available to stabilize the ankle. *Ankle arthroscopy* has transformed ligament surgery. Performed through tiny incisions, arthroscopy allows a fiber optic camera to be placed inside a joint. With minimal invasiveness, an injured area can be visualized and repaired. The ankle is "tightened" and instability eliminated. The "scope" procedure also cleans out ankle debris, scar tissue, and if necessary, removes and repairs injured ankle cartilage.

Caitlyn opted for the ankle arthroscopy, and a procedure called a *Brostrom-Gould* was performed. This surgery is highly effective for repairing damaged ligaments and restoring ankle stability. Caitlyn has now returned to all activities and even wears high heels again. Although she is no longer a competitive gymnast, Caitlyn can still do some pretty mean cartwheels!

How do I prevent sprains?

If you are a chronic "sprainer," seek professional help to evaluate your ankle. Therapy with a focus on strength, balancing, and mobility exercises under the care of a therapist can provide significant help. New procedures may also be available to return your ankle to as good as new in many cases. As I mentioned in Chapter 5, "Fun and Games," treating yourself like a professional athlete is a good way to avoid injury. Most professionals tape their ankles to provide extra stability and prevent twists and turns that lead to sprains. If you have repeatedly sprained an ankle, wear a brace for extra protection. Make sure your athletic shoes are sport specific; many injuries can be avoided by wearing the right footwear.

There are ankle injuries that you can't be prepared for, protect against, or avoid. The heel of your shoe breaks or you don't see the curb or you slip on a patch of ice. Accidents happen, but please get a specialist to evaluate any ankle injury!

My ankle is stiff and painful, and I don't recall injuring it. Could it be arthritis?

The ankle joint is a common location for arthritis. Like arthritis in the knee and hip, ankle arthritis has many causes, the primary ones being prolonged wear and tear, and a history of injury. X-rays reveal when there is arthritis in or around the ankle joint. There are a number of options for relieving discomfort and improving the function of the ankle. See Chapter 17, "Arthritis: A Joint Venture," for a detailed discussion of treatments for ankle arthritis, and take the first steps toward getting your foot and ankle partnership working again.

Tender Tendons

Many tendons course around the ankle and are vulnerable to stress and overuse. If you feel a new pain in your ankle and foot, it is likely to be a tendon speaking up. Too much work with too little rest can irritate a tendon and cause it to get inflamed. This is basically what tendonitis is—inflammation of a tendon.

Early recognition, diagnosis, and treatment are essential to returning your tendon to normal function. Continued and repetitive stress on an inflamed tendon can advance the damage from tendonitis to a dysfunctional and even a completely ruptured tendon, oftentimes requiring surgical repair. So listen to your complaining ankle and don't wait to get it looked at. A podiatrist can give an accurate diagnosis followed by a treatment plan to give that tendon the care and support it needs to heal.

Why did I get a stressed tendon?

Having tendonitis is pretty common, and foot specialists treat tendonitis on a regular basis. All types of people can suffer from this condition, but here are some of the top causes.

Heredity

Having the genes for flat feet is a big factor in developing tendonitis. Flat feet make the job of muscles and tendons harder to do, and this extra work, day in and day out, often means a tendon becomes strained. If you were born with this type of foot, you may have a tender tendon in your future.

Extra Pounds

Many of us put on a few pounds as we get older, and carrying that extra weight can overload your tendon and also cause your arches to flatten out.

Athletic Injury

Athletes in training or competition often overdo activities that strain ankle tendons. It is one of the more common sports injuries we treat and can cause competitive athletes to miss a significant part of a season.

Sudden Increase in Activity

You don't have to be an athlete to overuse tendons. Many simple everyday scenarios can cause tendonitis in the ankle area. Vacations with lots of walking or all-day shopping trips, if you are not used to them, can give you the same tendon trouble as a star athlete.

Shoes

Wearing summer sandals, flip-flops, slip-on flats, and shoes that offer little or no support can stress a tendon. Remember feeling good is more important than looking good.

Work

Are you standing or walking on hard surfaces at your job forty or more hours a week? Your tendons may let you know they are not happy about it.

The inside of my ankle hurts, is swollen, and I'm having trouble walking.

Pain and fatigue on the inside of the foot, arch, and ankle may be signs that your *posterior tibial tendon* has gotten cranky. This tendon runs along the inside of the ankle and attaches to multiple locations on the inside of the foot. I refer to this tendon as the arch "holder-upper" because it works hard to maintain and support your arch. It performs other jobs as well, such as providing strength to lift the foot when walking. When the tendon is overworked it can refuse to do its duties.

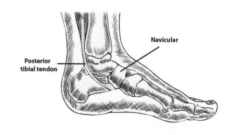

Evelyn, a patient at our practice, came in when her tendon went on strike. She limped into the office, complaining that she couldn't go grocery shopping or walk any distance without her foot getting tired and painful. She noted it had been getting worse over the last three months, and finally she had given up on the foot improving on its own and decided to have it looked at. Evelyn is sixty-eight and admitted to putting on about an extra 40 pounds over the last few years. Her left foot had a collapsed arch as compared to the right foot. When examined, her tendon was painful and swollen on the inside of the foot and ankle, and also noticeably weaker. On standing, Evelyn could balance on her good foot and do a one-legged toe raise, but on her left foot, she could not raise her heel up off the floor because the tendon was too weak and painful.

After evaluation, Evelyn was diagnosed with tendonitis of the posterior tibial tendon. Treatment was begun and included a special brace to wear, anti-inflammatories, and physical therapy. Thankfully, the tendon was not torn, and she was able to recover completely.

What are some home treatments for tendonitis?

Just like for a sprain, begin home treatment with RICE—Rest, Ice, Compress, and Elevate. Resting is often the most challenging element of RICE. Even if you stop exercising or playing sports, a normal day still requires lots of steps and movement. This makes it difficult to completely rest the tendon.

What treatments can podiatrists offer for tendonitis?

The staples of healing an injured tendon include reducing the workload of the tendon, elimination of swelling in the tendon, and finally strengthening the tendon. Extra support is usually provided through strappings, tapings, braces, CAM walkers, and orthotics. Anti-inflammatory treatments, physical therapy, and injection therapy are all additional treatment options along with the supportive therapy. Custom orthotics (specialized foot supports) worn in sports and daily shoes usually bring relief to individuals who have suffered from tendonitis, especially posterior tibial tendonitis. Your foot specialist will recommend the best plan to resolve the tendonitis and also offer remedies to prevent the tendon from flaring up again.

Evelyn, who you will remember came to the office after a few months of tendon trouble, has fully recovered, and she proudly reports she feels better than ever. She now wears her orthotics in all shoes and never goes out without them. She says the orthotics feel great and they give her arches and feet terrific support. The best news is they also will help prevent recurrence of her tendonitis.

My patient Carol was not so lucky. She lived with a posterior tibial tendon injury for over a year, hoping it would go away. But instead of getting better, it caused her increasing pain and trouble walking. She was stoic, but that didn't help her tendon. When she finally came to our office, after a year of suffering, her foot and ankle had completely collapsed. An MRI showed that the tendon was torn. Attempts to immobilize and then rehabilitate the tendon were unsuccessful. Carol had what is called *Stage 4 posterior tibial tendon dysfunction.* She went on to surgical repair in which the foot was realigned and a tendon transfer was performed to repair the tendon. After a significant recovery period, Carol is now walking without pain. But what should have been a relatively short route to healing an inflamed tendon turned out to be a long and difficult road for Carol because she put up with her painful tendon for too long.

I have pain along the outside of my ankle. Could it be a tendon?

There are two tendons that course along the outside of the ankle and extend into the foot. They are called the *peroneal tendons*, and they can become strained from overuse, injury, or gait abnormalities. If you have any pain running along the outside of the foot or ankle, peroneal tendonitis is a likely culprit.

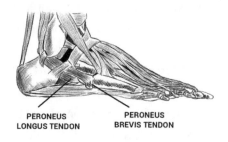

PERONEUS
LONGUS TENDON

PERONEUS
BREVIS TENDON

What causes peroneal tendonitis?

The most common causes of peroneal tendon injury are overuse and a sprained ankle, which can stretch the tendon and cause it to inflame. Runners and athletes also commonly injure this tendon. Curt Schilling's famous bloody sock of the 2004 World Series was the result of pitching too soon after surgery performed to repair a peroneal tendon injury.

Sometimes in a severe ankle sprain, the peroneal tendon is responsible for pulling off a piece of the bone it attaches to on the outside of the foot. This is called an *avulsion fracture.* This fracture may go unnoticed because the usual ankle x-rays do not focus on that part of the foot. It is often diagnosed later when the ankle is feeling better but the foot remains painful.

What are the treatment options for peroneal tendonitis?

The standard treatments for tendonitis discussed earlier are usually successful for relieving pain in the peroneal tendons. Patients who follow the care plan of a foot specialist can expect a return to normal activities.

I have numbness and shooting pain in my ankle and foot—tarsal tunnel syndrome?

When the nerve running along the inside of the ankle, known as the *tibial nerve*, is either injured or entrapped, it can cause shooting pains that are quite severe and debilitating. Patients with this condition, known as tarsal tunnel syndrome, also may feel numbness and a constant ache. You may have heard of carpal tunnel syndrome, which is a similar condition affecting the wrist and also caused by a pinched or irritated nerve.

What causes tarsal tunnel syndrome?

The tibial nerve can give you trouble for a number of reasons. Tight ligaments and structures around the nerve can cause it to become entrapped. Excessive pronation, or rolling in of the feet, often irritates the nerve. A direct injury to the inside of the ankle may damage the nerve and also leave you with chronic pain.

How will a podiatrist diagnose the condition?

Tarsal tunnel syndrome is often a challenge to diagnose. Because nerve injuries do not show up on x-rays, MRIs, or ultrasound, podiatrists make a diagnosis based on symptoms and an examination. Sometimes they use a specialized nerve test to support or confirm diagnosis. These tests, called *electromyography (EMG) and nerve conduction velocity (NCV) studies*, are helpful, although not always definitive.

Diane, a patient from Canada, experienced this difficulty in diagnosis firsthand. Diane traveled to our office in the Hudson Valley because she thought she might need cryosurgery to cure her severely painful foot. She had been diagnosed with plantar fasciitis; however, all treatments had failed, and her pain worsened to the point she could barely walk. She had researched cryosurgery as a possible treatment for plantar fasciitis. After a phone consultation, she made the trip to visit us.

When we evaluated Diane in our office, we discovered that, although there was evidence of plantar fasciitis, Diane's severe foot pain was due to tarsal tunnel syndrome. A branch of her tibial nerve was entrapped as it entered the foot. This is a form of tarsal tunnel called *Baxter's nerve entrapment* or *distal tarsal syndrome.* No wonder the common treatments for plantar fasciitis did not offer her relief!

Cryosurgery was attempted as it often can improve tarsal tunnel symptoms; however, when the pain continued, it was necessary to perform a special surgery to release Diane's entrapped nerve. Her pain was finally relieved and her life restored.

What are the nonsurgical treatments for tarsal tunnel syndrome?

Some patients, like Diane, will need surgery to relieve their symptoms, but not all patients. Treatment of tarsal tunnel syndrome may be as simple as wearing custom orthotics that minimize ankle rolling (pronation) and pressure on the nerve. Periodic injections, anti-inflammatories, and physical therapy may also be effective options for controlling pain from an injured or entrapped nerve.

Are there consequences for just living with tarsal tunnel symptoms?

Diane's story had a happy ending, and surgery does often bring relief to patients, but severe nerve damage can leave a patient in chronic pain and may not be repairable. If you suspect or have been diagnosed with tarsal tunnel syndrome, it's best to seek treatment sooner than later, as delaying treatment may make this condition more difficult to resolve.

Staying Up

Your ankles can go through lots of twists and turns over your lifetime. One thing we know for sure is that to have a happy foot you need a healthy ankle. The best way to be both happy and healthy is to ensure your foot and ankle always remain the dynamic duo they are meant to be. So, the next time your ankle slips up or goes sideways seek professional care from your podiatrist. We are here to make sure you and your ankle stay in full swing and always get a kick out of life.

Chapter 16

Broken Toes:
Let's Set Them Straight

You are most likely to break a toe in your home. That is where many of us let our toes roam barefoot and fancy-free. Unfortunately, bare toes are also exposed to dangers like couch legs, chairs, and beds. Pinky toe fractures are actually called "bedpost fractures" because ramming them on a bedpost is one of the more common ways to break a pinky. How many times has your toe had an encounter in the night with an unseen or forgotten obstacle? And what do most of us do about these injuries? A scream and a few choice words are often the limit of how we address a bashed toe.

I am going to let you in on something—broken toes should be treated. There is a commonly held belief that there is nothing anyone can do for a broken toe. I am sure you have heard this or maybe even said it yourself. But it isn't true! Broken toes can and should be treated because ignoring them often leads to trouble in toe town.

A Toe Story

I want to introduce you to Megan. She came into my office recently complaining of a painful toe, and her story, unfortunately, is one I hear so often I think I should share it with you.

Megan's second toe was permanently bent at the knuckle, a hammer toe. All her other toes were normal and straight. X-rays confirmed the hammer toe and showed arthritis in the joint. When I was taking Megan's history, I asked her if she had ever had an injury to that toe. She said no. But then remembered she did hurt her toe about a year before when she hit it one night on the bed frame. "Does that count as an injury?" she asked me.

Megan had decided at the time that at worst she might have broken the toe, but she didn't have time to have it x-rayed, there wasn't anything anyone could do for it anyway, and it would heal by itself. Well, guess what? That stubbed toe was an injury. In fact, it was a broken toe, and it could have been treated so Megan didn't end up with a painful, bent, and arthritic toe that needed to be corrected surgically! There you have it—a cautionary toe tale.

How can I tell if my toe is broken?

You can't. Unless it has dramatically changed position, you cannot tell if a toe is broken by looking at it. A toe fracture is extremely painful. It immediately swells and changes color to a nice black and blue, which indicates internal bleeding around the injury. But the only way to diagnose a broken toe is with an x-ray.

Won't a broken toe just heal on its own?

The body will work to heal any bone fracture (a fracture is a break). But if the broken bone is no longer in alignment, the toe may heal in a crooked or deformed position. This can cause long-term pain and swelling. That's why broken legs and broken arms are x-rayed—to see if there is a break and to reposition the bone if needed, making sure it will heal in the correct position to recover full function and be pain-free. And that is why broken toes should be x-rayed as well.

What happens after my toe is x-rayed?

The specialist will determine if your toe is fractured and if it needs to be realigned. Most broken toes do not need to be reset, just like most broken arms do not need to be reset. If your toe does need to be repositioned, a simple local anesthetic is placed in the toe before manipulating it back into its proper position for healing.

The x-ray also tells the foot specialist if the fracture goes through a joint. The second, third, fourth, and fifth toes have three bones and two joints each. If the toe fracture extends into a joint, this leads to a stiff, nonbending toe that over the long term develops arthritis. The earlier the toe is evaluated the better the prognosis and the less chance of arthritis arriving and settling into the toe.

The last piece of information the x-ray yields is the location of the break. Some locations heal uneventfully with time and simple treatment, while a bad break through a joint needs more medical attention and care. There is just no way to know without an x-ray. So please, if you stub your toe and see stars, and it gets swollen and black and blue, have the toe seen by a professional.

Can I go to the podiatrist for x-rays?

All podiatrists take x-rays, and most offices have same-day emergency care appointments. It is worth checking your local office. A visit to a podiatrist may save you time and get you seen by a specialist right away.

What can I do at home to help my broken toe?

As with many foot injuries rest, ice, compression (taping or wrapping), and elevation all should help to minimize swelling and pain.

How will the podiatrist treat my broken toe?

After x-rays are taken and the extent of the injury is evaluated, your podiatrist often places a splint on the toe. Foot specialists all have their own favorite splint or wrapping to help heal broken toes. Frequently, the fractured toe and its immediate neighbor are strapped together in a buddy splint. If the fracture is displaced, the toe will be reset after the toe is numbed with a local anesthetic.

What kind of shoe should I wear while I heal?

Sometimes a surgical shoe is needed to allow for pain-free walking. For simple toe fractures, a comfortable shoe suffices. Usually a wide shoe with a stiff bottom is best. A flexible shoe allows for too much bending of the toe. But as with all injuries what works best for healing depends on the location, type of fracture, and how much swelling and pain the patient is experiencing.

I broke my big toe. Is that a more serious injury?

The big toe, also known as the great toe or *hallux*, is more difficult to break than the other toes. Its two bones, the *proximal phalanx* and the *distal phalanx*, are both bigger and stronger than the bones of toes two, three, four, and five. This is because the big toe bears more weight when we stand and walk. That larger role makes breaking the big toe a more serious injury than other toe fractures. To off-load weight bearing, a broken great toe usually needs to be placed either in a surgical shoe or a CAM walker boot. On occasion, a great toe fracture can need surgical correction to limit painful arthritis and deformity.

Do I need to worry about a cut I got when I bashed my toe?

A cut on the toe when a break is also suspected is serious. This injury needs medical attention. A fracture with bleeding is considered an open fracture, and antibiotics are routinely prescribed to minimize any chance of a bone infection, or what is called *osteomyelitis*.

What about my toenail? It was injured when I broke my toe.

A broken toe may also be accompanied by an injury to the toenail. This is especially common when the toe gets jammed in a head-on collision with an immovable object. A toenail can be lifted off from the trauma, or there can be bleeding under the nail, which is called a *subungual hematoma*. This is most painful, and if there is a broken toe with a bloody nail, the nail is usually removed and the patient placed on antibiotics. In addition, any open wound needs evaluation for a tetanus shot if the patient is not up-to-date.

How can I prevent broken toes?

Wear shoes in the house, have a nightlight in your bedroom, and—I know this sounds silly—secure your frozen foods. All podiatrists have treated countless fractures from frozen food falling out of the freezer with a bull's-eye on your barefoot toe. A direct hit from hard, heavy frozen food can break or even crush a bone into many pieces. A crush fracture is called a *comminuted fracture* and can resemble a jigsaw puzzle on x-rays; however, with proper care Humpty Dumpty can be put back together again, almost like new.

For the Record

You now know a suspected toe break is not to be treated casually. Seek professional advice and care, starting with an x-ray. Although many broken toes heal without issue, many create long-term problems, such as hammer toes and arthritis, if not given proper attention. Remember to ice, elevate, and wrap your toe until a professional can see you. I hope the record has been set straight on broken toes, and if ever needed, your broken toe is set straight as well!

Chapter 17
Arthritis:
A Joint Effort

R emember the old folk song about bones that many of us sang as kids? "The toe bone connected to the foot bone. The foot bone connected to the ankle bone"? Well, that song had it right—all of our bones are connected. Anywhere two bones happen to meet in our body is a joint that connects the bones and allows for mobility. Toes bend, ankles bend, knees bend, hips bend, and joints are what ensure all that bending action is easy, fluid, and pain-free.

But joints can be sabotaged by an unwanted visitor. Arthritis may pay a call and prevent your joints from performing their role as connectors, making them inflamed, stiff, painful, and difficult to bend. When arthritis strikes any of the thirty-three joints of the foot, it can put the brakes on your daily routine. If arthritis in your feet is taking the flexibility out of life, don't stand for it. Explore treatments for getting your joints on the bend again.

What does arthritis do to joints?
To understand how arthritis affects a joint, you will first need to know how a healthy joint works. So let's take a tour.

Inside a joint, we have the ends of two or more bones coming together but not touching. The end of each bone is covered by a glistening, white, protective cap of *cartilage*, and the gap between the bone ends is called the *joint space*. The *joint capsule* forms a sleeve around the joint (the bone ends and joint space) and has a layer called *synovium* that produces joint fluid. This *synovial fluid* acts as a lubricant between bones and keeps the cartilage healthy. The cartilage, the joint space, and the joint fluid provide for a pain-free, healthy joint.

Now let's take a look at a joint with *osteoarthritis* (*OA*), which is the most common type of arthritis. In OA, the joint space narrows and the bone ends begin to rub against each other. This causes wear and tear on the cartilage, which over time becomes damaged and worn down, eventually leading to the joint becoming bone on bone. By the time this happens, pain, swelling, and stiffness have set in, along with decreased joint function and mobility.

OA can also be caused by an injury that has damaged a joint. In fact, injuries account for 10 to 15 percent of OA cases. When you think of all the joints we have in our feet (thirty-three in each foot) and all the times they have been damaged over a lifetime, it isn't surprising that many of us end up with arthritis in a joint or two.

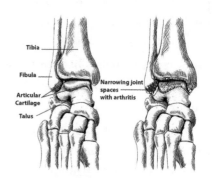

Rheumatoid arthritis (*RA*) is the second most common type of arthritis. RA is an autoimmune disease that can damage joints anywhere in the body and often affects the feet. The immune system normally protects the body, but in an autoimmune disease, the system mistakenly attacks the body instead. In RA, the immune system attacks the joint capsule, causing inflammation and damage to cartilage that can progress to the bone. RA also weakens the muscles, tendons, and ligaments surrounding the joint, which can lead to collapse of the joint. Science has no answer for what causes autoimmune diseases, but heredity seems to be one factor.

How do I know if I have arthritis and what kind it is?

When you first feel an aching, swelling, stiff, or painful joint, it is important to see a specialist. Don't dismiss the symptoms. Early detection and treatment can save your joint from becoming more arthritic and painful over time.

Believe it or not, medical literature identifies over 100 different forms of arthritis caused by diseases, conditions, or injury. The two we see on a regular basis in our office are osteoarthritis and rheumatoid arthritis, so I have concentrated on those here, but treatment is available to help manage all types of arthritis.

Osteoarthritis is diagnosed by evaluating your symptoms, x-rays of the joint, and clinical examination. A podiatrist most frequently makes the diagnosis of osteoarthritis in the feet, while an orthopedist makes the diagnosis of osteoarthritis in knees, hips, and other joints that may be causing pain.

Rheumatoid arthritis, on the other hand, is most commonly confirmed by a rheumatologist after completing a physical examination, blood testing, and a medical history. RA turns up in patients at younger ages than OA, appears in multiple joints (often symmetrically, meaning on both sides of the body), and runs in families. Past trauma to joints does *not* cause RA to develop. RA in its early stages can be difficult to distinguish from other types of arthritis, which all have similar symptoms, but please know it is essential to diagnose as soon as possible to limit devastating changes and joint destruction. Treatment with proper medications can help you avoid recurrent flare-ups and RA attacks.

Does everyone eventually get osteoarthritis?

No. Some people are much more susceptible to osteoarthritis than others. There are many influencing factors that can cause OA to develop. I'll ask you some of the questions I ask my patients when evaluating their risk factors for OA.

Do you work in the concrete jungle?

If you stand and work on hard concrete floors day after day, year after year, your joints may be talking to you. Your feet, ankles, knees, and hips are all subject to arthritis from the cumulative stress of years working on hard surfaces. Working in retail, on a factory floor, as a prison guard, mechanic, or contractor, or in any physically demanding job can be the reason you end up with arthritis in your feet. Sometimes in our office, we have to have difficult conversations with our patients when continuing in their jobs will mean suffering long-term consequences to their joints.

Who's your daddy (and your mama)?

Inherited traits like shape and flexibility of a joint, and general foot type (high arch, normal arch, low arch) all factor into the equation of whether you get arthritis in your feet. Feet that have rigid high arches tend to stiffen and develop arthritis over time. Flat feet with collapsed arches can also lead to early OA as excessive stress is placed on the weight-bearing joints.

Have extra pounds been sneaking up on you?

If so, those pounds may be putting pressure on joints, which often leads to pain and arthritis. Losing weight helps your health in many ways, including easing joint pain in hips, knees, and especially feet. Start a life change in your eating habits, and feel the difference it makes to your joints!

Did your foot and the bedpost ever meet in the night?

Think back. All of the bumps, twists, turns, sprains, and breaks you have experienced from run-ins with furniture, falls, sports, and car accidents are risk factors for arthritis. If some of those foot injuries have gone untreated, years later they may show up as arthritic joints. Muscles, tendons, and bones usually heal uneventfully, but a damaged joint is difficult to heal. An injury to a joint can erode the cartilage, leading to bone-on-bone rubbing and arthritis.

That's what happened to my patient Matt. Matt is thirty-one and a motorcycle enthusiast. He came to the office complaining that his foot didn't turn in or out like it used to and that it was so stiff and painful he was having a hard time walking.

When asked about past injuries, Matt said he had had a few spills on his motorcycle and some broken bones. The worst fall was the one that broke his heel bone five years before. The break had been a difficult one to heal, and the doctor treating Matt at the time had warned there might be some arthritis down the road. Sure enough, his x-rays now showed advanced arthritis throughout the back portion of his foot and heel bone. The arthritis was making it difficult for Matt to work. Because the trauma-related arthritis had become so advanced, Matt needed surgery to fix his foot and eliminate his pain.

Where am I most likely to get osteoarthritis?

Any joint can develop osteoarthritis, but podiatrists see OA most frequently in the big toe joint, the midfoot, and the ankle.

Why the big toe?

Arthritis around the big toe joint (medically known as the *first metatarsal-phalangeal joint*) is commonly caused by either injury or repetitive stress. The big toe has a big job as it propels us forward. Each and every step places full weight-bearing stress on the joint, which makes developing wear-and-tear arthritis in the big toe joint extremely common. Hereditary factors may also cause arthritis. For example, if your big toe joint happens to be squarer in shape, you are more likely to get arthritis in the joint than if it has a round shape. Square

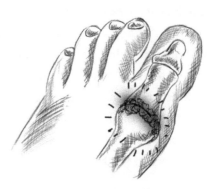

Great toe joint arthritis

joints are just stiffer and cause more wear and tear to cartilage. But don't feel too jealous of your friends with round toe joints. They are more likely to get bunions.

What is the treatment for arthritis in the big toe?

A podiatrist uses x-rays to confirm a diagnosis of arthritis in the "great," or big, toe joint. Depending on the severity, treatments can be anywhere from simple conservative options to surgical correction.

My patient Dot has been a waitress for the last twenty years. When she first came to see me four years ago, she complained of pain in her big toe joint. I saw she wore a fitness tracker, and I asked her how many steps she took each day. She said she averaged about 15,000 steps daily.

X-rays of Dot's foot showed a narrowed joint space with arthritis inside the big toe joint, plus large bone spurs on top of the joint, typical of wear-

and-tear arthritis. Dot takes an occasional day off to rest her foot. To relieve inflammation, she ices her foot and applies topical pain relievers. She switches her shoes often and wears custom orthotics. And when the pain is very acute, she comes to the office and receives a cortisone injection in her big toe joint. Dot is hoping to retire in a few years, but if the arthritis worsens, she may require surgery before then.

I tried the conservative treatments, but my big toe is still painful.

If pain in your arthritic big toe continues despite conservative treatment, or the arthritis progresses to an advanced stage, called *hallux rigidus*, your podiatrist may recommend surgery. When it comes to joint surgery, doctors often say, "When you are ready, let us know." Our job is to help you enjoy a good quality of life. If you cannot enjoy the activities you want to because of pain, then it may be time to consider surgical correction.

Most weeks I will see a patient who comes in after years of treatment and says, "Doc, I think it's time." In the winter, we typically fix golfers who want to be ready for golf season, and in the summer, we often correct painful feet for our skiers and teachers.

What are the surgical options for arthritis in the big toe?

For less severe arthritis in and around the great toe joint, recommended surgery often consists of a "cleanup" of the area. A common procedure removes bone spurs around the arthritic joint. Called a *cheilectomy*, this surgery can decrease pain from the bone-on-bone rubbing.

For more advanced arthritis, the procedure of choice is often a *fusion*. A fusion puts the two bone ends of the toe joint together into one, eliminating the arthritic joint and thus permanently relieving the pain. After a successful fusion, patients usually resume all normal activities without restriction. Another option is to have an implant placed in the great toe joint to separate the arthritic bone ends. Your podiatric surgeon will make the best recommendation based on your individual case to help relieve your pain.

Postcards from Darlene continue to remind me how rewarding what we do is for our patients. She suffered from increasing arthritis in her great toe joint before finally relenting and taking the time to surgically fix her joint. Darlene had been an avid hiker and world traveler, which is why she was so hesitant to have her surgery. She was worried it would limit her adventures. For many years now, I have received postcards from all over the globe, sent by Darlene while on her winter skiing trips and hiking expeditions. Each said, "Having a wonderful time—thank you, Dr. Tumen." The fusion procedure relieved her pain and allowed her to return to an active lifestyle. So take action today and don't let your big toe cramp your style.

My ankle is stiff. How do I know if it is arthritis?

Like the big toe joint, the ankle often develops OA. If you are having trouble walking or getting out of bed because of a stiff or swollen ankle, or you are now able to predict the weather by how painful your ankle is, it's time to have your joint checked out. X-rays of arthritic ankles often reveal bone spurs, narrowing of the joint space, and in advanced cases, bone-on-bone contact.

What are some treatments for ankle arthritis?

Sometimes patients use several treatments in combination or, as in my patient Fred's case, one after another as symptoms intensify. Fred is seventy-two and comes to the office regularly with his daughter for foot care. He has been a self-professed workaholic throughout his life with lots of manual labor. One of his primary complaints has been ankle pain caused by a history of many sprains and injuries. Fred's x-rays showed a complete lack of joint space with advanced arthritis.

At every appointment, Fred's lovely daughter asks him if his ankle hurts and if he wants a shot today. He unfailingly has a funny comment and wants to know why it doesn't get better. At first, cortisone injections worked well for Fred's pain, but the amount of relief began to diminish. He is adamant about avoiding ankle surgery until he absolutely can't walk any longer. I recommended a special ankle brace called an *AFO* (*ankle-foot-orthosis*). The custom brace is successfully stabilizing Fred's joint and decreasing his ankle pain. The brace and an occasional cortisone injection are doing the trick for Fred, at least for now.

But who knows, a new technology for repairing or growing new cartilage may be available before Fred needs to have surgery. Several exciting developments are currently in the works. So stay tuned for treatment advances by keeping in touch with your podiatrist.

What are the surgical options for an arthritic ankle?

The simplest surgeries for ankle arthritis remove bone fragments and bone spurs. These are often the result of prior injury. A bone spur can restrict motion and cause pain in and around the joint. Removing bone spurs can free up movement and reduce pain.

Ankle Arthroscopy

Arthroscopic ankle surgery is a preferred procedure for relieving mild to moderate arthritis. This surgery is performed through two small incisions. A tiny surgical instrument with an attached high-tech camera is inserted through one of the small openings. The image is magnified and viewed on a television monitor and shows any damage to the inside of the joint. Through the other opening, a surgical instrument attached to vacuum suction removes arthritic debris, damaged cartilage, small and medium-sized bone spurs, and scar tissue. Recovery from arthroscopic surgery is faster and easier than traditional surgery.

Ankle Replacement

For severe, painful arthritis that has failed all conservative treatments, ankle replacement is an option now helping many. Knee and hip replacements have long been a staple for these arthritic joints, but the ankle is a complicated joint and has previously proven difficult to replace. New improved implants are now making ankle joint replacements a more successful technique for those with severe ankle arthritis.

Ankle Fusion

Fusion is another option reserved for severe ankle arthritis. Ankle fusion removes all damaged cartilage, eliminates the joint, and combines the three ankle bones into one. Removing the painful joint relieves the pain permanently. Following a fusion of the ankle, motion is restricted, and the body compensates by other joints taking on more of the workload. It is important to ensure the joints surrounding the ankle are not arthritic, as they may take on added stress following fusion.

I have rheumatoid arthritis in my feet. How can my podiatrist help?

Treatment for painful rheumatoid feet varies depending on the person's pain, age, health status, and ability to walk. Conservative treatments such as cortisone injections can work well for controlling symptoms. My patient Martha is a great example of successful cortisone use. Martha is seventy-five and has RA that affects the joints in the middle of her foot. She comes into the office about every six months because of a flare-up. Her foot becomes painful and swollen on top, which makes walking and shoe wearing difficult. Martha usually requests a cortisone shot, and her swelling and pain go away and stay away for about another six months.

There are different medications available to help minimize painful arthritic attacks. Repetitive rheumatoid attacks can weaken and deform a joint or multiple joints. Special inserts and custom orthotics are commonly used to support, protect, and relieve pain from the rheumatoid foot. Sometimes custom shoes are needed to accommodate changes in foot shape.

With the advances in medications that limit rheumatoid flare-ups, it is less common for feet to become severely deformed these days. If surgery does become necessary it is usually isolated to a specific joint for pain relief. In the rare case of a severely deformed and painful rheumatoid foot, surgical reconstruction can be performed to reduce pain and restore function. Experienced foot surgeons can work wonders for those who suffer with painful RA.

How do I pick a surgeon?

How to choose a foot surgeon is discussed in detail in Chapter 20. All surgeons are not created equal, and selecting a skilled foot surgeon is crucial for success. Here, let me remind you that board certification, routine performance of the procedure you are having done, recommendations from staff, positive word of mouth in your community, and happy patients are all good indicators of a skilled surgeon.

Making the Right Connections

Arthritis pain can vary from a simple nuisance to a life-changing debility. If you are educated about your condition, your medical team can work with you to provide the proper treatment, support, and guidance to help navigate this challenging condition. Make managing your arthritis a joint venture and keep your foot happily connected to your ankle bone.

Chapter 18

Diabetes and Your Feet: Time to Team Up

Hearing your doctor say that you have diabetes can be overwhelming. Unfortunately, it is becoming a more and more common diagnosis. In 2012, over twenty-nine million Americans were living with diabetes, and it's estimated that double that number are currently prediabetic. The good news is that if you are diabetic or prediabetic, there is much you can do to improve your health status and prevent complications.

Many risk factors for diabetes are within your control. It may not feel that way because lifestyle changes are usually required and can be the hardest to make. But I have seen diabetic and prediabetic patients turn their lives and their health around. Most of them did not do it alone; they put together a team of doctors, nutritionists, exercise coaches, and loved ones to help them move steadily away from diabetes and toward a healthy lifestyle.

Diabetes can have a number of serious complications, but one many diabetic patients most fear is having a foot or leg become compromised by the disease. I will tell you what I tell my patients: if both of us do our part, we can dramatically lower the risk of that happening. But this means you must take responsibility and become the star player on your health team. Don't let diabetes dominate. Get educated about your condition, put together a winning strategy, and act on it.

What is the difference between Type 1 and Type 2 diabetes?

Type 1 diabetes, previously known as *juvenile-onset diabetes,* is usually diagnosed in childhood or adolescence. The exact cause of this type of diabetes is unknown, but it is believed to be an autoimmune response in which the body's immune system mistakenly attacks itself. In Type 1 diabetes, the immune system destroys insulin-producing *islet cells* in the pancreas. Insulin is required to allow glucose (the fuel the body makes from food) to pass into all of our body's cells. Without insulin, cells are deprived of energy, and cell function is impaired.

Type 1 diabetics experience a rise in their blood sugar levels because glucose is not being delivered into the cells. In order to provide the body's cells with energy and keep glucose from building up in the blood, Type 1 diabetics must receive daily doses of insulin either by injection or through a pump.

Type 2 diabetes, formerly referred to as *adult-onset diabetes*, is the result of many factors that over time cause the body to become insulin resistant. The pancreas may still produce insulin; however, the ability of insulin to help glucose enter the body's cells to fuel them decreases. Cells are not sufficiently nourished, and glucose (sugar) levels in the blood elevate. Patients in early stages of insulin resistance are diagnosed as prediabetic. Complete insulin resistance can and often does develop, leading to a diagnosis of Type 2 diabetes.

What are the factors leading to Type 1?

Because we don't understand what triggers the autoimmune system's attack on the insulin-producing islet cells, we don't know how to prevent it. There is some link to family history, but it has also been suggested a virus may be the root cause. However, the incidence of Type 1 diabetes remains level, with no increase or decrease in the percentage of people being diagnosed.

What are the factors leading to Type 2?

In a nutshell, eating the wrong foods and too much of them. Diabetes is becoming epidemic because of changes in the American diet. With the rise of fast food, processed foods, bigger portion size, and the significant increase in sugar and carbohydrates in our diet, our bodies have become overwhelmed and oversized. We are putting our bodies, our most finely tuned machines, under so much stress they can no longer function properly. Call it a mechanical breakdown. Imagine running your car on only two cylinders. As America's diet has transformed, we have too! We have gained weight and have consequently seen a meteoric rise in Type 2 diabetes.

Here's a peek at what's going on inside your body when you eat excessive amounts of food and too many foods with sugar. Food and sugar trigger your pancreas to release more insulin. The insulin tells your cells to take in glucose (the fuel made from the food you eat). At some point, the cells, which are not in need of any more glucose, reject the insulin signals. Your cells essentially say, "Enough already!" and eventually ignore the signal and start to become insulin resistant. The basic function of insulin to regulate blood sugar and provide energy to the cells is reduced or shut down, and you are on your way to a diagnosis of Type 2 diabetes.

What can I do at home to prevent or treat Type 2 Diabetes?

If you are prediabetic or even diagnosed with Type 2 diabetes, there is much you can do. What is needed is a return to a healthy lifestyle. Less fast food, less processed foods, less intake of sugars and carbohydrates, more nutritious foods, and more exercise. Educate yourself, and try these tips to set you on the road to a healthier life:

- Read and understand food labels. Know what a portion size is, how many calories are in it, and what percentage of good ingredients it contains, like fiber, protein, minerals, and vitamins.
- Reject unhealthy foods and don't keep them in the house.
- Decrease portion size.
- Cook more.
- Avoid fast food.
- Eat more vegetables.
- Decrease intake of sugar, carbohydrates, and soft drinks.
- Exercise.
- Surround yourself with others who care about your health.

It is possible to lose 10, 20, 30 pounds, or more with just sensible lifestyle changes. Don't be afraid to seek your physician's help. And it is possible to restore your body to healthy metabolic function and to become less dependent on pharmaceuticals. It can be done. It's never too late. Every day committed to a healthy lifestyle is a day where the burden placed on your body is decreased. Day by day, new habits can be created, new choices can be chosen, and a future of reduced risk and a healthy body draws nearer.

Will diabetes affect my feet?

That depends a great deal on you. Diabetics over time are vulnerable to two important risk factors: decreased circulation and deteriorating nerve endings in the feet. Both endanger the diabetic foot and create increased risk for foot ulcers and infection. But if you are educated about your condition, watchful for changes in your feet, committed to keeping appointments with your podiatrist to have your feet evaluated, and faithfully follow your foot specialist's instructions, you need not develop foot complications.

Also always remember that the best way to minimize risk is to keep your blood sugars under control. Checking your hemoglobin A1C every three months is the best test to monitor control of your diabetes. The closer to normal, the less likely you are to develop long-term systemic complications. It has been proven that an educated diabetic who maintains strict control has less chance of complications arising from their diabetic disease. You are the most valuable player in maintaining healthy feet!

How do I know if my circulation is impaired?

One sign may be having to stop and rest when you walk because of pain in your calf or legs. If you can walk only a short distance without pain, you may be experiencing a significant reduction of blood flowing to your legs and feet, a condition called *intermittent claudication*. There are many other signs of poor circulation, medically known as *peripheral arterial disease* (*PAD*), including loss of hair on your toes, feet, or legs; dry and scaly skin; thinning and shiny skin; discoloration of the feet; cold feet; and cramping leg muscles in bed.

What should I do if I think my circulation is poor?

Visit your podiatrist or primary doctor to have your circulation evaluated. The most important test to check circulation takes just seconds. There are two pulses in each foot; one on the top, the *dorsalis pedis pulse*, and one on the inside of the ankle, the *posterior tibial pulse*. If these pulses are easily felt and are normal, then circulation flowing to your feet is usually good.

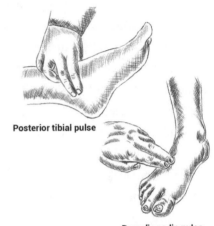

Posterior tibial pulse

Dorsalis pedis pulse

If your pulses are not palpable or if you have other signs of circulation impairment, the podiatrist refers you to the vascular doctor for further testing and evaluation. A simple noninvasive vascular test using blood pressure cuffs can give an accurate status on the amount of blood flowing to your feet. This test also helps determine if there could be a blockage constricting blood flow.

What can I do to help increase my circulation?

1. *Don't smoke.* A diabetic should never smoke. Smoking increases the risk of circulation disease, heart disease, and diabetic complications. If you are a smoker, seek guidance from your physician about a cessation program that will be safest and most successful for you.

2. *Exercise.* A simple twenty-minute walk on a regular basis works wonders to maintain your health and keep blood pumping to your feet. If the circulation is at all deficient, walking regularly helps your body maintain or improve circulation by developing what is called *collateral circulation*. This means your body creates new channels of blood flow to get around areas of poor circulation. Collateral circulation can take place in the legs and feet as well as around the heart. Exercise is one of the keys to avoiding diabetic complications. Walking is the easiest of exercises to do, so no excuses, start your walking program today!

How will I know if I have lost feeling in my feet?

You may not know and that's a real issue. The loss of feeling in the feet due to diabetes, called *diabetic neuropathy*, is a major risk factor for the diabetic foot. When a patient has diabetes for many years with blood sugar levels that are consistently elevated, diabetic neuropathy often develops. Slowly, nerve endings may start to lose the ability to feel certain sensations. In many cases, the neuropathy can come on so gradually, patients may not even be aware of how much sensation has been lost. This makes periodic evaluation by a doctor of utmost importance.

Your podiatrist, primary care physician, or endocrinologist checks for neuropathy with simple in-office tests. A fine wire, called a *Semmes-Weinstein* monofilament wire, is used to determine if your nerve endings still maintain normal nerve sensation. If you can feel the fine wire with your eyes closed on all the locations of your foot, your protective sensation is intact. If you cannot pass the fine wire test, you may 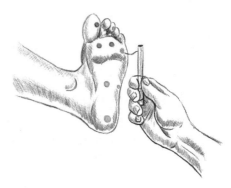 be at increased risk for developing a diabetic foot ulcer.

Does loss of protective sensation in my feet mean I have poor circulation?

These are two separate and distinct complications. It is essential to understand diabetic neuropathy can be present, and the feet can still have normal circulation.

Why is loss of protective sensation a risk factor?

When a diabetic's nerve endings are losing their natural ability to feel, this is called, *loss of protective sensation*, or *LOPS*. It's called that because feeling is a protection, and without it you are vulnerable.

The consequences of a loss of sensation can be quite serious as our patient John found out. John is fifty-eight, diabetic, and a chef who must stand on his feet for long hours. When he took off his shoes and socks after his shift one night, he saw blood on his sock. That's when John began to wonder if something was amiss. A week later when he finally came to our office, his foot was swollen and red, and had a foul odor. He also had a fever and was not feeling well. You guessed it. John's foot was infected.

What caused the infection? It turns out John had a splinter. He had stepped on a piece of wood, but did not feel the splinter enter his foot. Because he had neuropathy, there was no "Ouch!" moment. And without that ouch, he did not know to look at his foot. As the days went on and John worked on his feet, he was unaware that anything was wrong until he saw the blood on his sock. Without sensation in his feet, John was not protected.

I have limited sensation in my foot, but it's painful.

Diabetic neuropathy usually starts gradually. It is most often symmetrical (occurring in both feet) and frequently begins in the toes and works its way through the foot. Sometimes there is just numbness, sometimes there is tingling and burning, and sometimes it can even become painful. Yes, a numb, diabetic foot with neuropathy can become painful. This is called *diabetic painful neuropathy*, or *DPN*.

DPN can be quite severe and affect a person's ability to sleep, walk, maintain employment, and enjoy a normal quality of life. Often different medications or other treatments become necessary to attempt pain relief, allow for sleep, and to decrease burning, which may be so extreme it feels like your feet are on fire.

What is a diabetic foot ulcer?

If you are a diabetic with neuropathy or poor circulation, you are vulnerable to developing a wound on your foot. These wounds are called *diabetic foot ulcers* (*DFUs*). It is estimated that up to 15 percent of diabetics develop a foot ulcer at some point in their lifetime. Healing of a diabetic foot ulcer can be challenging and depends on the size and depth of the ulcer, presence of infection, quality of the circulation, and whether bone is involved. It is imperative for the patient to comply with all doctor instructions to successfully heal foot ulcers. A foot ulcer that does not resolve can put a foot at risk.

Remember our patient John? The one who got a splinter in his foot that he did not feel? That splinter caused an ulcer, which then became infected. After his foot was examined at our office, John was immediately placed in the hospital. He had surgery to drain the infection, intravenous antibiotics, and an extended home stay—out of work and off his feet—to eventually heal the diabetic foot ulcer. John's foot was saved because he had excellent circulation.

After this experience, John understands that he has advanced diabetic neuropathy and is at risk for additional diabetic foot ulcers. In the future, he will inspect his feet daily, not go barefoot, and keep regular appointments with our office. John now has shoes that protect his feet, which he wears with special inserts. These provide extra cushioning to safeguard his feet from the excessive pressures of the concrete surfaces he works on. He also promises that at the first sign of any problems, he will seek medical care immediately.

What can I do to avoid foot ulcers?

The majority of diabetic foot ulcers start in the front part of your foot around the toes or the ball of your foot. These areas take extra weight-bearing pressure with walking and also become irritated by shoes that rub on bony prominences, such as hammer toes or under the metatarsal bones. A podiatrist can evaluate your foot for likely pressure points. For example, a corn on a toe, a callous on the ball of the foot, a thickened toenail may be subject to excessive pressure, irritation, or possible infection. These may seem like small issues, but for an at-risk diabetic, they can quickly escalate into a dangerous ulcer.

Susan is a diabetic patient who learned that lesson the hard way. She came to the office with an excruciatingly painful corn between her fourth and fifth toes. She explained that she worked at a bank and wore dress shoes every day to work. During the exam, we saw that the area was red and swollen, and that there was a red streak running up her foot. The corn was more than just painful, it was now an infected ulcer. We placed Susan on antibiotics, had her infection cared for, and had the corn reduced. Once Susan was healed, we performed a small surgical procedure on her hammer toe to prevent the corn from returning and the diabetic foot ulcer from recurring.

If Susan had come in to see us for a checkup or when she first had symptoms, she could have avoided the ulcer and the infection. During a checkup, we can identify any risk areas on the foot and protect them. Cushioning, special inserts, better shoes, corrective procedures can all help prevent ulcers. Prevention is especially important if you have neuropathy and may not be able to feel when a spot on your foot begins to rub. A list of more things you can do to protect your feet follows.

More Tips for Proper Care of the Diabetic Foot

- Inspect your feet daily.
- If you cannot see the bottoms of your feet, use a mirror or have a family member inspect them for you.
- Make sure there are no cracks or openings in the skin.
- Moisturize daily, best to get a recommendation for a moisturizer brand from your doctor.
- Avoid being barefoot. Wear shoes to protect your feet.
- Schedule an annual checkup with your podiatrist.
- At every primary care visit, take your shoes and socks off and have your physician check your feet, pulses, and evaluate for neuropathy.
- Wear shoes that fit well, have room for your toes, and are wide enough to prevent rubbing and irritation.
- Avoid over-the-counter corn and callous removers.
- Check water temperature before bathing, especially if you have any signs of neuropathy.
- Avoid hot tubs.
- Wear socks with good cushioning.
- Avoid shoes without socks to prevent blisters and irritations.
- Ask your podiatrist about special shoes. Medicare and other insurances have special programs that pay for shoes and inserts for at-risk diabetics.
- Walk. It is the best exercise to keep circulation flowing.
- Keep your blood sugar levels as close to normal as possible.
- Do not smoke.
- Find a good podiatrist, and put him or her on your diabetic team.
- Educate yourself on diabetes. Seek a hospital or community group that offers diabetic education seminars.
- At the first sign of a foot problem, call your podiatrist. Never wait to see what happens.

- Love your feet.
- Keep them for life.

Don't Be an Ostrich

An ostrich is known for burying its head in the sand. Podiatrists often feel some of their diabetic patients behave the same way. They bury their heads and ignore their diabetic disease.

So many of the devastating diabetic foot complications are avoidable, but these complications remain on the rise. Too often diabetics avoid the necessary steps to minimize risk factors. What's even more frustrating is when a diabetic lives with a foot ulcer for an extended period before seeking treatment.

Meet Albert. He works as an auto mechanic, is in his sixties, and showed up at our office with a severe diabetic foot ulcer that he had been ignoring for over a month. He had continued to work and did not seek medical care until he became really sick with a high fever and his foot and leg became red and swollen. When he was asked why he left it so long, he simply stated: "I didn't want to lose my foot, and I was afraid it may have to be amputated."

It is my experience that the reason so many diabetics put off treatment for foot ulcers is fear. The fear is a foot ulcer leads to amputation. So patients who know they have a wound avoid seeking treatment because they are afraid the doctor may tell them they could lose a toe, or a foot, or a leg. Of course, the opposite is true. The sooner the specialist treats a foot ulcer, the better chance the patient has of minimizing risk of a devastating complication. Come in at the first sign of trouble. Don't hide from your ulcer or from your podiatrist.

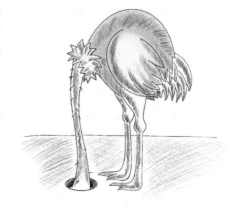

And just so you know, podiatrists don't always give out bad news to diabetics. It is so gratifying to have diabetic patients come in for an annual exam and leave happy because they had a good checkup. Lighten your load of worries, see us annually, and let us prevent, protect, and put a smile on your face.

You Can Do It—Just Like Barbara and Joe

Taking a stand and changing habits is not easy, but it is possible to trade in your one-way ticket to diabetes for a healthier lifestyle and a happier future.

I want you to meet Barbara and Joe, two patients who are winning the fight against diabetes and obesity after making an unexpected decision to take action. Married more than forty years, Barbara and Joe had always looked forward to retirement. But when retirement came, it was not at all how they had imagined it. Over the years, obesity had crept up on them. With a combined weight of about six hundred pounds, walking had become difficult and their lifestyle more and more sedentary. Diabetes and painful arthritic joints were just two of the health issues they were coping with. It looked like Barbara and Joe could only look forward to sharing bigger and bigger health challenges.

Then, it happened. They finally got "fed up." Their joints and everything else hurt, they could barely leave the house, and they saw their doctors more than their grandkids. They decided it wasn't too late for them, and diabetes and other weight-related problems would not control their future. They started to change their lifestyle. They consulted a dietician and now meet with her regularly to learn about nutrition and get help planning healthy meals. They began exercising and take a walk together every day. They supported each other in making these lifestyle changes.

Amazingly, in just under a year, Barbara and Joe have lost a person between them—over 200 pounds. Blood sugar levels are returning to normal, and their medication has been decreased. Their joints hurt less, and they can play with their grandkids again. They are now getting healthier, having more fun, and looking forward to their future—together. What a pleasure to see them so happy and motivated to get more out of their golden years. If Barbara and Joe can do it, so can you.

If you are ready, go for it! Gather a team, include healthcare professionals and loved ones, and publicly declare your goals of changing your lifestyle. Make a plan. Write it down. How much weight do you want to lose? What are you going to do for an exercise plan? Who is going to support you? Who is going to join you in a wonderful lifestyle change? Make your next meal a healthy one. Start today!

Chapter 19

Gout:
A Royal Pain

"Grace, can you please squeeze me in today?" When the phone rings at the office and Grace hears Charlie's voice, she knows immediately he is having another gout attack. Charlie has been a patient for years and, unfortunately, has suffered many episodes of gout during that time. He averages a gout attack about once every six months or so, and usually he has a story about a business lunch with clients, indulging in foods or alcohol that he knows he should have avoided. When Charlie shows up sheepishly at the office, he typically has a painful, red, hot, swollen great toe joint, and he can't even put his shoe on.

Many people think of gout as an old-time ailment. Not an unreasonable assumption given that we have accounts of gout going back centuries, and many illustrious names on the historical list of sufferers. Both Charlemagne and King Henry VIII are thought to have had the condition, as well as Benjamin Franklin, who chronicled his experience in *Dialogues between Franklin and His Gout*. Unfortunately, gout is not a thing of the past; it is very much with us today. In fact, it is estimated that between five and eight million Americans currently are afflicted with this condition.

People with gout experience "attacks," in which a joint becomes very painful. Gout attacks often come on suddenly and sometimes seemingly without cause. They are usually so excruciating the sufferer seeks the nearest doctor's office, urgent care, or emergency room. Many people with gout end up at a podiatrist's office because 50 percent of gout attacks are in the big toe joint. Any experienced podiatrist has handled numerous cases of gout and developed a go-to plan both for offering relief and managing the condition.

Who gets gout?

Although women are not spared, a majority of patients with gout are middle-aged men. One possible reason for gout favoring men is their tendency to have higher uric acid levels. Women do become more prone to gout after menopause, even equaling men in rate of attacks.

What triggers a gout attack?

Gout is triggered by a buildup of *uric acid*. Like many substances, uric acid is normally found in the blood and performs an important job, which is protecting blood vessels from damage. Uric acid works as an *antioxidant* to clear *free radicals* from the linings of blood vessels. When there is too much uric acid in the blood, however, it forms crystals, officially called *monosodium urate crystals*. These sharp needle-like crystals get deposited in a joint, causing terrific pain and inflammation, with the joint becoming swollen, red, and warm.

Why do uric acid levels get too high?

Uric acid is produced when *purines* are metabolized to provide energy inside our cells. Our bodies naturally make purines, and some of the foods we eat may also contain high levels of purines. Our cells are not picky and use purines from both these sources, releasing uric acid into the blood as a by-product. The kidneys are in charge of regulating the amount of uric acid transported in the blood by eliminating some when there is too much.

But this system can get out of balance. The body can either make too much uric acid (overproduce) and/or remove too little uric acid (underexcrete). Both can cause the level of uric acid in the blood to become too high above normal, potentially causing a gout attack.

tests give the doctor a picture of the variation over time in the uric acid level and aids in the medical management of the condition.

X-rays

Not used as a primary diagnostic tool, x-rays can be helpful in revealing damage to the joint. The term *gouty-arthritis* is commonly used when x-rays show damage to the joint accompanied by painful symptoms of arthritis.

What are the treatments for gout?

When gout attacks, pain relief is the primary concern for patients. Doctors have many different ways to treat gout based on their experience in relieving a patient's pain. There is not one way to treat gout correctly. Treatments are geared for either relief of acute gout or to minimize future attacks. Let's start with acute gout.

Anti-inflammatories

The standard gout prescription is an oral anti-inflammatory, which reduces pain and swelling around the joint. There are many anti-inflammatories a doctor can choose from, although indomethacin is one of the most commonly prescribed. Relief is usually gradually obtained over a number of days.

Injection Therapy

In our practice, a corticosteroid injection has become the standard treatment for a painful gout attack. This is my go-to treatment because an injection gives the fastest pain relief, reduction in swelling, and return to shoes. A local anesthetic applied with the injection gives immediate pain relief, and the corticosteroid acts quickly to reduce painful symptoms within twenty-four to forty-eight hours. Also, because oral anti-inflammatories can cause stomach upset or other side effects, one simple injection relieves pain and mitigates the need for pills.

Colchicine

This medicine is also used for an acute gout attack. It is not known how colchicine works, but it is believed it suppresses the immune system. Although colchicine is a proven form of treatment for gout, it is not one I frequently use for my patients because of unpleasant and often severe side effects, such as diarrhea.

Oral Steroids

Prednisone taken orally is another treatment option. Doctors often prescribe a decreasing dosage pack called a Medrol dose pack.

Waiting It Out

Eventually, a gout attack dissipates on its own, even without treatment. This may sound tempting, but, here's the rub. In addition to extending the time you suffer with pain, the longer the joint stays inflamed, the more damage is being done. Enduring multiple extended attacks will eventually leave you with a permanently painful arthritic joint. So a word to the wise: toughing it out is not your best option.

What can I do to avoid future gout attacks?

No matter what the cause of your gout, dietary changes are a smart choice to defend against gout attacks. Now before saying "I don't eat or drink any of the things that cause gout," have an open mind and be honest. There are always tweaks you can make to your diet if gout is a big enough problem in your life. You may have no choice but to carefully watch everything you eat and avoid certain foods if you suffer from frequent gout attacks. For some, even straying once can cause an attack. So let's review.

Restrict Alcohol Intake

Not all alcohol has the same risk as far as gout is concerned. Beer is by far the biggest offender as it contains the highest concentration of purines of any alcoholic beverage. So if you suffer from gout, beer should be the first thing to go. Sorry, but someone has to be the bad guy. Hard liquor and spirits of all sorts are next on the elimination list if you suffer from gout. For those in need of some form of alcohol, there is good news. To date, studies have not implicated wine as a trigger of gout.

Avoid Fructose

A common ingredient in sodas, fruit juices, sports drinks, and many food items, fructose has been shown to elevate uric acid. Avoiding fructose is important for minimizing gout attacks. High fructose corn syrup (HFCS) is an especially damaging form of fructose and a serious health risk for many people, including those with gout.

Don't Eat Foods High in Purines

Foods high and moderately high in purine content are listed below. Eliminating these foods from your diet helps to keep uric acid levels from elevating. Just like all types of alcohol are not the same when it comes to purines and maintaining normal uric acid levels, neither are all foods. Dairy products are usually lower in purines and safer for those with severe gout. When in doubt, consult a registered dietician for guidance.

Foods Highest in Purine Content

- Anchovies
- Game Meats
- Herring
- Mackerel
- Scallops
- Brains
- Gravies
- Liver
- Sardines
- Sweetbreads

Foods Moderately High in Purine Content

- Asparagus
- Beef
- Bullion
- Chicken
- Crab
- Duck
- Halibut
- Kidney Beans
- Lentils
- Lobster
- Mussels
- Bacon
- Bluefish
- Cauliflower
- Clams
- Dried Beans and Peas
- Goose
- Ham
- Lamb
- Lima Beans
- Mushrooms
- Mutton

- Navy Beans
- Oysters
- Perch
- Shrimp
- Turkey

- Oatmeal
- Peas
- Pork
- Spinach

Do Eat Foods and Drink Fluids Low in Purines

Even though the lists above seem quite long, there are many healthy foods to enjoy. First, remember to drink plenty of water. Water is healthy and keeps you hydrated, which benefits your blood. Fruits and many vegetables are not implicated in gout so enjoy them too. Dairy products and low-fat foods are also on the safe list.

Prescribe Yourself Some Cherries

In addition to foods that don't raise your uric acid level, there are foods that can actually help lower it. Tart cherries contain compounds helpful in minimizing both gout and arthritis. A frozen concentrate of cherry juice is a good source.

Shed Extra Pounds

Dropping excess weight has been shown to reduce gout attacks. So here is yet another motivation to get out and start walking. Lose weight and lose your gout. Not a bad deal!

What if diet changes are not preventing my gout attacks?

It is the goal of most physicians to help you control your gout with dietary changes alone. Neither doctors nor patients want to rely on long-term use of medicines. However, repeated gout attacks are not only painful, they also may increase the risk of developing arthritis in the various joints under attack. So if conservative treatment is not helping, your doctor may prescribe medication to lower uric acid levels, prevent gout attacks, and protect joints.

I have chronic gout, what are my risks and options?

If you suffer from chronic gout, make sure you meet with your primary care doctor for testing to help understand causes. Your doctor may also have new medications that may help you avoid attacks, so keep in touch.

Frequent gout attacks over years can have consequences. These include the development of chronic arthritis and also the formation of *tophi*. Tophi are soft tissue lumps that form from excessive uric acid crystals in afflicted joints. Like snowflakes, a few uric acid crystals don't amount to much, but many crystals packed together take on heft—think of a snowball, only smaller. Tophi vary in size from a small pea-sized lump to the largest I have encountered, which approached the size of a golf ball. The toes are a common place for tophi to develop. Although they are not necessarily painful, it is not unusual for the tophi to become irritated by shoes, and possibly cause an infection. If necessary, tophi can be removed, although there is always a chance of more developing.

Don't Go Down in History

Even though the list of gout sufferers is full of history's rich and famous, you don't want to add your name to it. Now that you know all about the gout, see your podiatrist and get the gout out!

Chapter 20

Surgery: What You Need to Know

S urgery is a serious commitment. There are always risks and no guarantee of success. The foot has an intricate and complex design. That means small changes can have big consequences, for better or worse. In our practice, we only recommend surgery as a treatment option to relieve foot pain, to improve foot function, or to repair a foot deformity—in other words, when it's worth it.

That said, with our ever-growing understanding of biomechanics plus improved technologies, foot surgery is becoming less invasive, less painful, and more successful all the time. In my thirty years of practice, there have been extraordinary advances in surgical procedures for some foot conditions, returning a highly functioning, pain-free, and good-looking foot to the patient! But getting a great result depends on two people—your surgeon and you. That's why a serious commitment is necessary. Your part is to commit to following instructions, and your surgeon's part is to commit to helping you get the best outcome possible.

Not all foot surgeons are created equal. This is a hard truth, and it means, of course, that you have to figure out whom to entrust with your foot. Not all patients do due diligence in selecting a surgeon. Either they don't understand the importance or don't know what to look for or ask. So in this chapter, I offer some tips for finding the right foot surgeon and getting the best result for your foot.

Should my surgeon be board certified?

Board certification is available in every medical and surgical specialty. In podiatry, the certifying surgical board is the American Board of Foot and Ankle Surgery. Although certification is not a guarantee of a great result, you can be assured that the surgeon possesses the necessary skills required for successful foot and ankle surgery. For more information, visit abfas.org.

Should my surgeon be a podiatrist or an orthopedist?

As a patient, you want to find a surgeon who specializes in foot surgery. That means the surgeon performs foot surgery every time he or she enters the operating room. The occasional foot surgeon is not usually a great foot surgeon. So, whether a podiatrist or an orthopedist, what matters is that your surgeon is all about the foot.

I know so many great foot surgeons who live, breathe, and love foot surgery. It is their life. Most are podiatrists. It is just my world. The orthopedists who *only* perform foot surgery are also skilled foot surgeons. The great majority of orthopedists, however, do not specialize in foot surgery. They operate on knees, hips, shoulders, the spine, and more.

We live in a world of specialization. Podiatrists spend on average seven years specializing in the foot and ankle before going into private practice. An orthopedist specializing in foot surgery usually does a one-year fellowship in foot and ankle surgery after residency.

This does not mean I recommend all podiatric surgeons unreservedly. As in any profession, there are great podiatric surgeons and not so great. You just want to find the most competent and experienced surgeon available to perform your foot surgery.

What to Ask

When choosing a surgeon, you should ask questions. Although it may feel uncomfortable, any good surgeon is happy to answer all your questions to help make you comfortable prior to surgery. Coming in with a list is a fine idea. Remember the saying, there are no silly questions, only silly answers.

About the Surgery

You need to feel confident that your surgeon is competent and skilled at the procedure recommended to fix your foot. That means in addition to being board certified, they should perform the particular procedure you need regularly. Here are some questions to ask about the surgery:

- What is the name of the procedure you are going to perform?
- How often do you perform this surgery?
- What is the most common complication from this procedure?
- What type of anesthesia is used?
- Where do you perform the procedure—in an office, hospital, or surgical center?
- What result do you expect from the surgery?
- What are the other surgical and nonsurgical options for my condition?

About Postsurgery

Patients often underestimate the importance of care after surgery. In our practice, we commonly see patients one week after surgery, two weeks after, and so on, until healing is complete and the patient returns to normal activities. Ask your surgeon about follow-up care. Make sure they are committed to seeing you through the healing and rehabilitation process and that you understand what is involved. Here are some example questions to put you and your surgeon on the same page regarding aftercare:

- How long will I be laid up?
- What are the postsurgical instructions to limit swelling and discomfort?
- How often will you see me after surgery?
- How long before I can wear a shoe?

- When can I drive?
- How long before I can exercise?
- When can I return to work?
- What will I need to do to support my recovery?
- Will physical therapy (PT) be necessary?

About the Costs

It's helpful to be prepared for the financial costs of surgery. Many surgeries are commonly covered; however, some may not be. Find out before the surgery so you can avoid surprises. Start by asking your surgeon and your insurance company these questions:

- Will insurance cover some or all of the procedure?
- Is my insurance accepted?
- What other associated costs may not be covered?
- Will follow-up care be covered?
- Will there be prescriptions?
- Will I need any devices, such as a post-op shoe, walking boot, or crutches?

Ask Around

Word of mouth is often the best way to find a good surgeon. Results matter! Talk to the staff in your surgeon's office. Speak to others in the waiting room. Satisfied or unsatisfied patients are happy to share what went right or what didn't. Ask your primary care doctor and other doctors and nurses in your community who they would recommend and why.

Is a second opinion necessary?

Who's to say the second opinion will be better than the first? The time for a second opinion is when you are not comfortable with the first opinion, the doctor, or office staff. Then, by all means, get another expert to give you advice. Also, if you are advised to have surgery and you do not want surgery, get another opinion.

Everyone has an opinion. Yours is the most important. Trust your instincts. You know when a surgeon is confident. When you do not get a great feeling, hold off on scheduling surgery and get another opinion. This is your foot; you get to choose who fixes it! If you have researched the surgeon, been satisfied by their answers, gotten a recommendation from others, and you are comfortable and confident—you should be good to go. Foot surgery can be a wonderful game changer for you, your foot, and your lifestyle. Here's to pain-free walking and wearing shoes comfortably!

Conclusion
How to Become a VP—Virtual Patient

know at this point in a book, a conclusion usually signifies the finish line. It wraps up loose ends, recaps main points, lets you take a nice deep breath of satisfaction, and then move on. But for this book, my hope is that we are now just at the start.

With in-office patients, "conclusion" is a word we don't often use. Once you are a patient at our practice, we consider you always our patient. Our office doors remain open for help and assistance. The same goes for this book. It is always available and open to you. Pick it up any time you have questions or concerns about your feet and ankles. The answer you seek is probably in here. But I want the book to be more than just a resource. I want it to be your invitation to a relationship.

As a patient, when you go to a doctor's office, you are put in a private room, the doctor comes in, and you get personal one-on-one time with him or her. Sometimes you wait too long, and sometimes you get too little time, but that is the system we are accustomed to, and for the most part, it works. You develop a relationship with a doctor. With a book, you can get information and learn, but my goal with *Ask the Foot Doctor* is that, if you want to, you can take the next step and communicate directly with us.

What I have learned over my thirty years in podiatry is that each person's foot problem is unique to them. This book will give you great answers and information, but sometimes, you will want to talk about your problem, ask more specific questions, and get personalized advice. Is this serious, should I be worried? Can I do something to get this to go away? How can I get rid of the pain the fastest?

At *Ask the Foot Doctor*, we are opening our virtual doors to you. You have a question, we want to answer it for you. Need advice, we want to help. Want a referral to a qualified foot doctor, we can get you hooked up. Want your own personal, private telemedicine consultation, we can make it happen!

Is this a big task? Maybe. But we are going to try because everyone needs a solution that is the best fit for them.

As I've mentioned in the book, no two feet are the same. That means in America alone there are over 680 million feet. Sometimes a customized solution is needed. Sometimes it just feels better to get trusted, personal advice to put a worry, a pain, or a challenge behind you.

When I wrote this book, I imagined just sitting and talking to one of my patients. I would write as if I was having a one-on-one conversation with that person. We want you to be able to talk to us too, and so we are taking that extra "step" for you. As the book title says: Ask the Foot Doctor!

If you would like to become a virtual patient, contact us and ask away. It's simple. Just send an email to *question@askthefootdoctor.com*. Now that we are virtually there for you, the last page of this book does not have to be our conclusion. It can be an opening to a new chapter.

It is my greatest wish that this book has provided value to you and your feet. That you can take this information and share it to help your family, your friends, and loved ones. My goal has been to help each person who picks up this book discover a way to move forward, keep in motion, take on a healthier lifestyle, or resolve a nagging foot issue. I hope it has done that for you.

If you would like to receive periodic updates on foot care recommendations, tips, as well as the latest in state-of-the-art advances, just email us at *info@ askthefootdoctor.com*. We will be happy to add you to our contact list and stay in touch. We will keep the foot facts coming your way.

For now, be kind to your feet, show them some love, and truly appreciate all they do for you! I am reminded of a quote I would like to share with you: He who has his health has a thousand dreams, he who does not have his health has one. Here's to good health, happy feet, and a lifetime of pain-free walking. And don't forget to stop by and visit us online at *askthefootdoctor.com*. See you there!

Fun Foot Facts

- Leonardo da Vinci was the first to create accurate anatomical drawings of the foot, and he called feet "a masterpiece of engineering and a work of art."
- Each remarkable foot contains 26 bones, 33 joints, 107 ligaments, and 19 muscles.
- There are a total of 250,000 sweat glands in both feet! The average foot produces about a half a pint of moisture daily.
- Sneakers got their name from their quiet rubber soles, which were less noisy than leather-soled shoes. This allowed the wearer to "sneak" up on others without being heard.
- Hippocrates, the Greek physician, is said to have been the first to study corns and calluses, and developed the first scalpels to remove them.
- An estimated 2.4 billion pairs of shoes are sold each year in the United States alone.
- Guinness World Records recognizes Darlene Flynn as having the largest shoe collection with over 14,000 different shoe-related items. Most women own an average of fifteen pairs of shoes.
- Women have about four times as many foot problems as men. Fashionable shoes and high heels are partly to blame.
- The average stride is 2.5 feet, so most of us take approximately 2,000 steps to walk a mile.

- The average person walks the equivalent of four times around planet Earth in a lifetime.
- At least 75 percent of Americans will experience a significant foot problem at some point in their lives.
- Madeline Albrecht was employed for fifteen years at Hill Top Research Laboratories, where her job was to sniff feet for the benefit of a better-smelling world. Madeline sniffed an estimated 5,600 feet and holds a Guinness World Record for this amazing feat!
- There are said to be more websites for foot fetishes than there are for foot health.

Acknowledgments

This book started as my dream and has been a work in progress for over three years. What I learned is that writing a book is a labor of love. Lots of labor, lots of love.

Of course, as in any venture, nothing happens without an amazing team. Each person is vital to the process and together magic can be made. So, here are the magicians who levitated me and helped make this book appear before your very eyes.

Three years ago, I had no idea about the vital role an editor plays in the process of writing a book. Now I do. In medical speak, your editor is your doctor. They doctor your words and breathe fresh air into them. I am most grateful to Kathy Rawson for her indispensable skills and commitment to this project. Our Friday meetings were a joy and they will be missed. Kathy has elegantly nurtured and transformed a medical manuscript into a welcoming and informative book. So now all who aspire to discover more about their feet can understand exactly what the doctor is saying without need of a translator. Thank you, Kathy!

Thank you to my brother, Michael Tumen. He has been my mentor and voice of encouragement for a lifetime. I followed in his footsteps into the world of podiatry and have relied on him for just about everything one can in life. I am grateful for having the best big brother a person could have. His patients are lucky to have such a caring doctor, and I am lucky to have such a great role model in my life.

Every person should have a guardian angel, and I have had one since I stepped into podiatry school in 1979. John Grady has been watching over me and has been there for me every step of the way. Hands down, he is the smartest, humblest, and nicest person I have ever met, and is an amazing leader in the field of podiatry. If you are near Chicago and need a foot doctor, he is your man. Thank you for all you do for me and everyone in your life.

My partners at Hudson Valley Foot Associates are extraordinary on so many levels. From great doctors to great friends, our practice has grown each year while overcoming the obstacles and minefields that any business has to navigate. We are successful for one main reason, we are all committed to our patients and providing only the highest-quality care to our community. Thank you to Mike Keller, Danny Longo, and Cliff Toback.

Thank you to my life partner, Jenna Knudsen, who brings the fun to each and every day. Your encouragement, humor, huge smile, unconditional love, and generous spirit are my source of energy and inspiration.

Thank you, Bud Walker, you are always there for support and guidance. Thank you to Daniel Wright and Amanda Maloney for your research. Thank you, Karen Anderson, for the jump-start to get this book to the next level, your guiding hand, and introducing me to my fabulous editor.

Special thanks to Alan Chartock, WAMC/Northeast Public Radio and Medical Monday. I am also grateful to the many who teach and encourage growth. Thank you to Jeff Walker for sharing how to have a greater impact; Joe Polish for helping create a 10x mindset; Tim Ferriss for inspiration; Noah Kagan for your down-to-earth wisdom, wit and 5:30 a.m. challenge; and Jeffery Combs for the importance of sitting your butt in the chair. Special appreciation to Mom, Dad and Sister. Mom for always seeing the good in everyone, Dad for giving me a great start, and Sister for always being there.

A huge thank you to the fabulous people at Morgan James Publishing. They have an amazingly dedicated team that has made publishing this book a joy from start to finish. It is such an awesome feeling to work with a sensational team who remove all roadblocks and pave the way to making your dream come true. Kudos to Morgan James Publishing!

As Helen Keller said: "Alone we can do so little, together we can do so much." I am grateful for the wonderful people who together, by adding both inspiration and expertise, helped to deliver this book from baby steps to the finish line.

About the Author

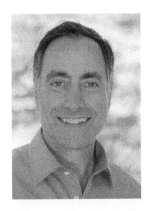

D
r. Tumen is a board-certified podiatrist with over thirty-five years of experience treating patients. He is a founding partner of Hudson Valley Foot Associates in Upstate New York. Dr. Tumen is a regularly featured guest on Northeast Public Radio's *Medical Monday*. He has published numerous articles for national magazines, newspapers, and medical publications. Dr. Tumen is an avid fitness enthusiast, having completed nine marathons, and is devoted to living and teaching a healthy lifestyle. He is a recipient of the Pride of Ulster County Award and also has served as Honorary Chairman of the Juvenile Diabetes Foundation Walkathon.

Shoes That Fit

It is a true pleasure to announce that proceeds from this book are being shared with Shoes That Fit, an extraordinary not-for-profit organization. Did you know that 1 in 5 American children are in desperate need of new shoes? Shoes That Fit has donated over 2 million pairs of new athletic

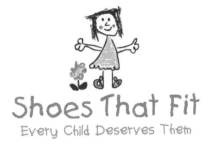

shoes and other necessities to children in need since 1992, helping over 120,000 children in 2017 alone. The mission of Shoes That Fit is to target one of the most visible signs of poverty in American by giving children in need new athletic shoes to attend school with dignity and joy, prepared to learn, play and thrive. The long-term goal is that no child should go to school with shoes that don't fit or cause foot pain. What a wonderful goal!

Here are some amazing statistics: Over 85% of schools teachers an 85% increase in self-esteem after students receive new shoes, 68% an increase in participation of physical activities, 39% higher attendance at school, and 54% report behavior improvement. All from a new pair of shoes. Please visit their website at shoesthatfit.org to learn more and discover how you can participate in helping children have shoes that fit! There's nothing better than helping a child.

Printed in the USA
CPSIA information can be obtained
at www.ICGtesting.com
JSHW082229140824
68134JS00017B/806

9 781642 791983